Copyright © 2024 Tessa Holloway
All rights reserved.

No part of this publication may be reproduced, distributed, or transmitted in any form or by any means, including photocopying, recording, or other electronic or mechanical methods, without prior written permission from the publisher, except for brief quotations in critical reviews and certain other non-commercial uses allowed by copyright law.

This book is nonfiction. The information provided reflects the author's research, experience, and knowledge at the time of writing. It is meant for informational and educational purposes only and is not a substitute for professional advice. The author and publisher bear no responsibility for any errors or omissions or for the consequences stemming from the use of this information.

Contents

Dedication and Acknowledgment	XI
Foreword	XIII
About the Author	XV
Introduction	XVII
1. Understanding Toxins in the Home	1
2. Creating a Non-Toxic Home Environment	9
3. Safe and Sustainable Living Practices	17
4. Navigating Product Labels and Certifications for Household Products	21
5. The Hidden Dangers in Your Home	25
6. Air Quality Matters	33
7. Detoxifying Your Kitchen	37
8. Water is Life: Ensuring a Safe and Sustainable Supply	47
9. Green Cleaning Basics	55

10.	Revamping Your Laundry Routine	59
11.	Non-Toxic Bedroom Bliss	63
12.	Living Room Liberation	67
13.	Bathroom Detox	71
14.	Decluttering for Health	75
15.	Safe Flooring Solutions	79
16.	Healthy Walls and Paints	83
17.	The Role of Plants in Detoxification	87
18.	Kitchen Pantry Detox	91
19.	Outdoor Spaces for Health	95
20.	Smart Technology Choices	99
21.	The Impact of Light and Sound	103
22.	Seasonal Detox Strategies	107
23.	Building a Non-Toxic Community	113
24.	Sustaining Your Toxin-Free Lifestyle	117
25.	Recipes for the Home: Cleaning Solutions	121
	Natural Pine Needle All-Purpose Cleaner	
	All-Purpose Cleaner	
	Glass and Mirror Cleaner	
	Non-Toxic Floor Cleaner	
	Natural Bathroom Scrub	

Wood Furniture Polish
Carpet Deodorizer
Toilet Bowl Cleaner
Dish Soap
Laundry Detergent
Oven Cleaner
Non-Toxic Brass Cleaner
Cleaning Chopping Boards
Disinfecting Wipes
Clean Drains
Mattress Cleaner
Non-Toxic Heavy-Duty Scrub

26. Personal Care and Skincare Recipes   135
Magnesium Spray (Relaxation and Muscle Relief)
DIY Lip Balm
Natural Body Butter
Non-Toxic Room Spray
DIY Deodorant
Non-Toxic Toothpaste
Natural Hand Scrub
DIY Hair Conditioner
Non-Toxic Essential Oil Shaving Cream
DIY Face Balm
Natural Body Scrub

Herbal Hair Care Shampoo
Natural Lip Scrub
Natural Deodorizer Spray
Face Wash for Acne
Herbal Salve
Non-Toxic Essential Oil Hair Conditioner
Non-Toxic Essential Oil Lip Balm
Non-Toxic Essential Oil Body Wash
Non-Toxic Whipped Lip Cream

27. Advanced Cleaning and Household Recipes   149
Laundry Bar Soap
Window and Stainless-Steel Cleaner
Sleepy Time Magnesium Butter
Homemade Infused Lavender Oil
Odor Eliminator Spray
Herbal Linen Spray
Disinfecting Spray
Toilet Cleaning Tablets
Non-Toxic Wall and Ceiling Cleaner
Non-Toxic Heavy-Duty Scrub
Rug and Carpet Cleaner
Non-Toxic Kitchen Cleaner and Deodorizer
Magical Sink Scrub
Homemade Laundry Detergent

Dishwasher Detergent
Non-Toxic Rinse Aid for Dishwasher
Non-Toxic Dishwasher Tablets
Non-Toxic Essential Oil Herbal Laundry Wash
Non-Toxic Essential Oil Herbal Laundry Softener
Non-Toxic Laundry Wash for Sensitive Skin
Non-Toxic Herbal Stain Remover
Non-Toxic Hand Wash
Non-Toxic Dish Wash
Non-Toxic Weed Killer
Non-Toxic Oven and Stove Solutions
Non-Toxic Home Appliance Cleaner
Non-Toxic Floor Cleaning
Keeping Your Home Smelling Clean and Fresh
Gentle Marble Cleaning

28. Lifestyle and General Wellness   169
Keeping Laundry Whites Bright
Cleaning Armpit Stains
Cleaning Grout and Shower Screens
Steam Cleaner and Squeegee for Cleaner Windows
Tincture Recipes
Non-Toxic Vapour Rub
Whipped Tallow Balm
Conquer Bug Season: Bug Spray

      Herbal Sleepy-Time Magnesium Butter

      Immune-Boosting Tincture

      Natural Energy Boost Tea

29. Conclusion   177

References   179

Dedication and Acknowledgment

Dedication

This book is dedicated to everyone working hard to build healthier, safer, and more harmonious homes. May it motivate you to adopt a toxin-free lifestyle and turn your living spaces into true sanctuaries of well-being.

Acknowledgments

This journey could not have happened without the unwavering support and encouragement from my family, friends, and the dynamic community committed to healthy living. I sincerely appreciate your motivation, which has inspired me to realize this vision. I extend special thanks to my editors and readers who have shared this journey with me. Your feedback and support have been essential.

Foreword

A TRULY *"CLEAN HOME"* encompasses more than its appearance; it's about guaranteeing that every breath you take, every surface you come into contact with, and every product you use contributes positively to your well-being. As synthetic materials and chemical-laden products proliferate alongside increasing environmental concerns, detoxifying your home has become more essential than ever.

This book acts as your handbook a call to action to rejuvenate the health of your living space and, consequently, your overall life. With practical advice, simple recipes, and actionable steps, we will embark on this transformative journey together to cultivate a home that not only appears clean but genuinely nurtures and enhances your well-being.

About the Author

Tessa Holloway is a talented author recognized for her insightful and engaging works that explore themes of personal development, independence, and the quest for a meaningful existence. Growing up in the lively coastal city of Sydney, Australia, Tessa quickly admired the beauty and resilience of nature. This bond with the natural environment fueled her enthusiasm for off-grid living, sustainability, and devising practical solutions for contemporary challenges.

With a foundation in environmental studies and extensive hands-on experience, Tessa infuses her knowledge and passion into writing books that inspire readers to lead more self-reliant and fulfilling lives. Her writings embody her strong conviction that everyone has the capacity to cultivate a more balanced and sustainable lifestyle, regardless of their starting point.

Tessa's path to authorship started with her passion for storytelling and a wish to impart practical wisdom. Her own experiences of adopting a simpler lifestyle, exploring remote areas, and learning from resilient communities inspired her. These experiences have crafted her distinctive viewpoint, which she incorporates into every page she writes.

When Tessa isn't writing, she likes to garden, explore nature, and try out DIY projects that reflect her dedication to sustainability. She also enjoys connecting with her readers and peers, frequently hosting workshops and engaging with communities excited to start their own journeys towards sustainability self-sufficiency.

Tessa Holloway seeks to inspire readers through her books to reclaim their independence, embrace significant change, and find joy in living harmoniously with nature. Her commitment to her craft and her audience establishes her as a credible voice in sustainable living and personal empowerment.

Introduction

Welcome to Home Detox Revolution, your comprehensive guide to cultivating a safer, cleaner, and healthier living environment for you and your family. In today's world, where hidden pollutants, chemicals, and toxins often permeate our homes, it's increasingly essential to take proactive measures to mitigate these risks. This book provides you with the knowledge and practical tools necessary to transform your home into a sanctuary for health and wellness.

This guide addresses your concerns about indoor air quality, the dangers associated with harsh cleaning agents, and the subtle repercussions of everyday household items. Your home should serve as a haven that nurtures both body and mind. However, contemporary living frequently invites unseen dangers, such as volatile organic compounds (VOCs), synthetic fragrances, and hazardous chemicals, into our daily spaces.

In this book, we'll assist you in identifying and removing these threats, presenting practical detox solutions and natural alternatives to establish a genuinely safe and healthy home. We'll delve into strategies for detoxifying your environment room by room, providing straightforward recipes and actionable advice to make your journey easier.

By making mindful changes and adopting sustainable practices, you not only safeguard your family's health but also contribute to a cleaner, greener future. Let this guide motivate you to take small, deliberate steps toward a home that nurtures both your well-being and that of the planet. Together, we can foster a healthier, more harmonious living environment for all.

Chapter 1

Understanding Toxins in the Home

What Are Indoor Pollutants and Toxins?

Indoor air pollution arises when toxic substances and pollutants build up inside the home, posing risks to the health and well-being of its inhabitants. Many of these pollutants are both invisible and odorless, rendering them hard to detect without specialized equipment. Despite this, their presence can greatly affect the indoor quality of life, particularly since people spend a large part of their time indoors. Below are some of the most frequently encountered indoor pollutants:

Volatile Organic Compounds (VOCs)

VOCs are gases emitted by household items and construction materials such as paints, varnishes, carpets, adhesives, and cleaning agents. Common VOCs include:

Formaldehyde: A recognized carcinogen found in building materials, furniture, and various household products, formaldehyde can cause respiratory irritation, headaches, and allergic reactions, especially in poorly ventilated areas.

Benzene: Commonly released from tobacco smoke, paints, and certain plastics, benzene has been linked to serious health concerns, including leukemia.

Toluene: Found in paint thinners, adhesives, and nail polish, toluene can affect the nervous system and cause dizziness, headaches, and irritation with prolonged exposure.

Phthalates

Phthalates are used as plasticizers in products such as vinyl flooring, shower curtains, and personal care items. They are linked to hormone disruption, respiratory issues, and reproductive health concerns. Extended exposure to these chemicals can have a more significant effect on children and pregnant women severely.

Particulate Matter (PM)

Particulate matter comprises small airborne particles like dust, pollen, and soot. Fine particles (PM2.5) pose specific risks since they can deeply infiltrate the lungs and reach the bloodstream, potentially causing respiratory and cardiovascular issues problems.

Biological Pollutants

These comprise mold spores, pet dander, dust mites, and bacteria. Biological pollutants flourish in damp or inadequately ventilated spaces, potentially worsening allergies, asthma, and other respiratory issues conditions.

Health Effects of Indoor Air Pollution

Indoor air pollutants can cause both immediate and long-term health issues. Knowing these risks allows you to take proactive steps to minimize exposure and protect your family's health well-being.

Respiratory Issues

Indoor pollutants such as volatile organic compounds (VOCs), formaldehyde, and particulate matter can irritate the respiratory system, causing symptoms such as coughing, wheezing, and shortness of breath. These impacts are especially dangerous for individuals with asthma or chronic respiratory conditions.

Allergic Reactions

Common allergens like dust mites, mold, and pet dander can cause sneezing, itching, watery eyes, and nasal congestion. Prolonged exposure may intensify symptoms and potentially result in asthma.

Fatigue and Headaches

Extended exposure to indoor pollutants such as formaldehyde and phthalates may lead to ongoing headaches, chronic fatigue, and a general feeling of discomfort, diminishing overall quality of life life.

Chronic Health Risks

Certain indoor pollutants like formaldehyde and phthalates are associated with greater long-term health hazards including:

Increased risk of cancer

Developmental problems in children

Reproductive health issues in adults

Children, older adults, and individuals with compromised immune systems are particularly vulnerable to the effects of indoor air pollution.

Sources of Indoor Toxins

Understanding where indoor toxins come from is the first step in eliminating or reducing them in your home. Below are some of the most common sources:

Building Materials

Products such as plywood, particleboard, and insulation often contain adhesives and chemicals that, over time, off-gas harmful toxins.

Furniture and Furnishings

Newly purchased upholstered furniture, carpets, and mattresses often release VOCs and may also contain flame retardants that degrade air quality.

Cleaning Products

Many standard cleaning products contain harsh chemicals and synthetic fragrances, which release VOCs and contribute to indoor air pollution.

Personal Care Items

Cosmetics, skincare products, and synthetic fragrances can contain phthalates, parabens, and other potentially harmful chemicals that contribute to indoor toxins.

Heating and Cooking Appliances

Gas stoves, kerosene heaters, and improperly vented fireplaces can emit carbon monoxide and nitrogen dioxide, both of which are harmful when inhaled.

Tips for Reducing Exposure to Indoor Toxins

Creating a safe and healthy indoor environment requires a combination of mindful choices and proactive practices. Here's how to tackle indoor toxins:

1. Choose Low or Zero-VOC Products

Choose low or zero-VOC building materials, furniture, and paints to reduce harmful emissions. Seek certifications such as Greenguard or Green Seal for assurance of safety standards.

2. Ventilate Your Home

Effective ventilation is essential for minimizing indoor pollutants. Whenever feasible, open windows and doors to promote fresh air circulation. Utilize exhaust fans in kitchens and bathrooms to eliminate moisture and maintain air quality pollutants.

3. Use Natural Cleaning Products

Switch to eco-friendly cleaning solutions made with safe ingredients like vinegar, baking soda, and essential oils. These alternatives are not only safer but also effective in maintaining cleanliness.

4. Avoid Synthetic Fragrances

Synthetic air fresheners, candles, and personal care products can emit harmful chemicals. Choose fragrance-free or naturally scented options made from essential oils.

5. Filter Indoor Air

Invest in a high-quality air purifier with a HEPA filter to capture airborne pollutants such as dust, pollen, and pet dander. Regularly replace HVAC filters to ensure optimal performance.

6. Reduce Dust and Allergens

Dust and vacuum frequently, using a vacuum with a HEPA filter.

Wash bedding, curtains, and soft furnishings regularly to remove dust mites and allergens.

Use dehumidifiers in damp areas to prevent mold growth.

7. Inspect and Maintain Your Home

Consistently inspect for mold, leaks, and structural damage that may contain pollutants. Resolve these concerns swiftly to ensure a safe living environment.

8. Go Green

Houseplants like spider plants, peace lilies, and pothos can help improve indoor air quality by absorbing certain toxins and increasing oxygen levels.

Taking Control of Indoor Air Quality

By pinpointing indoor pollution sources, recognizing their health implications, and applying these strategies, you can establish a safer, cleaner, and healthier home environment. The aim is to decrease toxin exposure and cultivate a space that enhances overall well-being for you and your family. Minor, regular adjustments can lead to substantial improvements over time, making your home a haven of health and comfort.

CHAPTER 2

CREATING A NON-TOXIC HOME ENVIRONMENT

CHOOSING ECO-FRIENDLY BUILDING MATERIALS and Furnishings

Establishing a sustainable and healthy home environment starts with choosing the right materials and furnishings. By carefully selecting eco-friendly options, you can minimize your environmental impact and improve indoor air quality and overall well-being.

Sustainable Materials

Sustainable Materials: Are environmentally friendly, durable, and visually appealing. Think about these options:

Bamboo Flooring: Bamboo grows rapidly and regenerates without the need for replanting, making it a renewable and sustainable flooring choice.

Reclaimed Wood: Using reclaimed wood for flooring, beams, or furniture gives new life to old materials while reducing deforestation and landfill waste.

Cork Flooring: Cork is harvested from the bark of cork oak trees without harming the tree, making it both renewable and biodegradable. It is also naturally resistant to mold and pests.

Recycled Glass Countertops: These countertops are made from post-consumer or industrial glass and come in a variety of colors and styles. They are durable, non-toxic, and highly sustainable.

Choose Non-Toxic Finishes

Traditional paints, varnishes, and sealants can emit harmful VOCs, which degrade indoor air quality. Instead, choose:

Low-VOC or Zero-VOC Paints: These options significantly reduce the emission of harmful chemicals. Brands often offer certifications like GreenGuard or EcoLogo to ensure safety.

Water-Based Varnishes: These provide a safer alternative to solvent-based finishes and are just as effective in protecting wood surfaces.

Select Natural Textiles

Synthetic fabrics often contain chemical treatments, such as flame retardants and water repellents, that release toxins over time. Opt for:

Organic Cotton and Linen: Free from synthetic pesticides and dyes, these textiles are breathable, soft, and hypoallergenic.

Wool and Hemp: Naturally resistant to moisture and durable, wool and hemp are excellent choices for upholstery, rugs, and curtains.

Avoid Flame Retardants

Numerous furnishings have dangerous flame-retardant chemicals associated with health problems like endocrine disruption and developmental delays. Search for products certified by organizations such as OEKO-TEX or GOTS (Global Organic Textile Standard) to guarantee they lack these toxins. Always review product labels and ask about chemical composition treatments.

Indoor Air Purification Techniques

Maintaining clean indoor air is essential for a healthy living space. Implement these techniques to improve air quality naturally and effectively:

Invest in Air Purifiers

High-quality air purifiers equipped with HEPA filters can capture up to 99.97% of airborne pollutants, including:

Dust and pollen

Pet dander

VOCs and smoke particles

To optimize their effectiveness, place air purifiers in high-use areas such as living rooms, bedrooms, and home offices.

Add Houseplants

Certain houseplants naturally filter toxins from the air while adding a touch of greenery to your home. Examples include:

Peace Lilies: Excellent for removing VOCs like benzene and formaldehyde.

Snake Plants: Known for converting CO2 into oxygen at night, making them ideal for bedrooms.

Spider Plants: Easy to care for and effective at reducing carbon monoxide and other toxins.

Boston Ferns: Great for adding humidity to dry indoor air while filtering pollutants.

Enhance Ventilation

Proper ventilation dilutes indoor pollutants and maintains air freshness.

Natural Ventilation: Open windows and doors regularly to allow outdoor air to circulate.

Mechanical Ventilation: Use exhaust fans in kitchens and bathrooms to remove moisture, smoke, and odors.

Whole-House Systems: Consider installing an energy-recovery ventilator (ERV) or a heat-recovery ventilator (HRV) for consistent airflow throughout the home.

Tips for Minimizing Exposure to Electromagnetic Fields (EMFs)

Electromagnetic fields (EMFs) from electronic devices are an often-overlooked source of indoor environmental stress. Reduce exposure with these strategies:

Limit Device Usage

Reduce screen time, especially before bed, to lower EMF exposure and improve sleep quality.

Encourage family members to engage in non-digital activities to reduce reliance on electronic devices.

Use Wired Connections

Replace Wi-Fi with Ethernet cables for internet connections whenever possible.

Use landline phones instead of cordless models to eliminate RF radiation.

Create EMF-Free Zones

Designate areas in your home, such as bedrooms, where electronic devices are not allowed. These zones:

Promote better sleep quality by minimizing electromagnetic interference.

Provide a space for relaxation and disconnection from digital distractions.

Strategies to Reduce Indoor Humidity and Prevent Mold Growth

Excess humidity fosters mold growth and contributes to poor air quality. Manage humidity levels effectively with these methods:

Use Dehumidifiers

Install dehumidifiers in areas prone to moisture, such as basements, bathrooms, and laundry rooms.

Maintain indoor humidity levels between 30–50% to discourage mold growth.

Repair Leaks Promptly

Regularly inspect plumbing, roofs, windows, and gutters for leaks.

Address any signs of water damage immediately to prevent moisture buildup.

Improve Ventilation

Use exhaust fans in kitchens and bathrooms to remove excess moisture.

Install ventilation systems in areas like attics and crawl spaces to enhance airflow and reduce condensation.

A Blueprint for a Non-Toxic Home

Adopting eco-friendly building practices, enhancing indoor air quality, reducing EMF exposure, and controlling indoor humidity are essential for achieving a healthier home. These approaches safeguard your family's health while supporting environmental sustainability. Implementing these strategies results in a living space that promotes well-being, lessens environmental footprints, and encourages a stronger connection to principles of sustainability.

Chapter 3

Safe and Sustainable Living Practices

Energy Efficient Home Practices

Reduce energy consumption: Adopt energy-saving habits such as turning off lights and unplugging electronics when not in use. Utilize energy-efficient appliances to minimize power usage.

Upgrade to energy-efficient appliances: Replace outdated appliances with Energy Star-certified models that consume less energy and reduce utility bills.

Enhance home insulation: Proper insulation in walls, floors, and attics helps maintain indoor temperatures, reducing the need for heating or cooling and improving energy efficiency.

Utilize renewable energy sources: Consider installing solar panels or wind turbines to generate clean energy. These systems can lower carbon emissions and decrease dependence on fossil fuels.

Waste Reduction Strategies

Recycling: Establish a home recycling system to sort materials like paper, cardboard, plastics, glass, and metals. Follow local guidelines and clean recyclables before disposing of them.

Composting: Create a compost pile or use a compost bin for organic waste like fruit scraps, vegetable peelings, coffee grounds, and yard trimmings. Composting reduces landfill waste and produces nutrient-rich soil for gardening.

Reduce single-use plastics: Replace disposable items such as plastic bags, water bottles, and utensils with reusable alternatives, such as cloth bags, stainless steel bottles, and bamboo utensils.

Water Conservation Tips

Fix leaks: Regularly check faucets, toilets, and irrigation systems for leaks and repair them promptly. Even small drips can waste significant amounts of water over time.

Install water-saving fixtures: Upgrade to water-efficient faucets, showerheads, and toilets that conserve water without compromising performance. Look for Water Sense-labeled products.

Practice mindful water use: Take shorter showers, turn off the tap when brushing teeth or washing dishes, and run full loads in dishwashers and washing machines.

Eco-Friendly Lifestyle Choices

Support local and sustainable products: To reduce the environmental impact of transportation, buy from local businesses and artisans. Prioritize products made from sustainable materials and eco-friendly production methods.

Practice mindful consumption: Focus on quality over quantity by repairing or repurposing items and avoiding impulse purchases. Choose products that align with your values and consider their environmental and social impact.

Reduce food waste: Planning meals, creating grocery lists, and properly storing food to extend its shelf life. Also, leftovers should be used creatively, and inedible food scraps should be composted to minimize landfill waste.

Incorporating these safe, eco-friendly practices into your daily routine can significantly reduce your environmental footprint, conserve valuable resources, and contribute to a healthier planet. By implementing small, intentional changes to your habits and lifestyle, you can collectively promote a more sustainable and resilient future for coming generations come.

Chapter 4

Navigating Product Labels and Certifications for Household Products

Understanding Eco-Labels and Certifications

Eco-labels and certifications: Are marks on product packaging indicating that a product adheres to particular environmental or sustainability criteria. Below are some widely recognized certifications to consider for:

Energy Star: Signifies that a product meets energy efficiency standards set by the U.S. Environmental Protection Agency (EPA). ENERGY STAR-certified products consume less energy and help reduce greenhouse gas emissions.

USDA Organic: Indicates that a product adheres to the organic standards set by the United States Department of Agriculture (USDA). Certified products are made with organic ingredients and are free from synthetic pesticides, fertilizers, and GMOs.

Green Seal: This symbol represents products that meet environmental and performance standards established by the non-profit organization Green Seal. These products are designed to be eco-friendly and safe for human health and the environment.

Cradle to Cradle Certified: Recognizes products assessed for environmental and social impacts throughout their lifecycle—from raw material extraction to disposal. These products emphasize sustainability and circularity.

Forest Stewardship Council (FSC) Certified: Ensures that wood or paper products come from responsibly managed forests. FSC-certified products support sustainable forestry practices and conservation efforts.

Tips for Deciphering Product Labels

Understand key terms:

Organic: Indicates the use of organic ingredients certified by a trusted body. Labels like "100% organic" or "certified organic" ensure compliance with organic standards.

Eco-friendly: Suggests minimal environmental impact during design, production, or packaging. However, this term is not regulated and may be used vaguely.

Non-toxic: This denotes the absence of harmful chemicals or toxins. To ensure safety, look for labels stating "non-toxic" or "free from harsh chemicals."

Spotting Greenwashing and Making Informed Choices

Greenwashing: refers to deceptive marketing practices falsely presenting a product or company as environmentally friendly. Here's how to identify and avoid it:

Look beyond marketing claims: Examine the product's ingredients, materials, and manufacturing processes. Don't rely on slogans or imagery alone.

Verify third-party certifications: For independent validation of environmental claims, opt for products certified by reputable organizations like ENERGY STAR, USDA Organic, or Green Seal.

Consider the entire lifecycle: Evaluate the product's environmental impact from sourcing and manufacturing to packaging, use, and disposal. Prioritize products designed for sustainability and circularity.

Support transparent brands: **Look for** companies openly sharing information about their supply chains, sustainability efforts, and environmental impact. Also, look for businesses that publish sustainability reports or detail their eco-friendly practices.

You can make educated purchasing choices by learning about eco-labels and certifications and how to read product labels and identify greenwashing tactics. These actions help you align your decisions with your values, lessen your environmental footprint, and back companies and products that are truly committed to sustainability.

Chapter 5

The Hidden Dangers in Your Home

Awareness serves as the primary defense in establishing a safe and healthy living space. Many common items in our homes harbor concealed dangers, including hazardous chemicals, pollutants, and unsafe materials. Although these threats may not be apparent at first, they can build up over time, presenting serious risks to our health and well-being. By recognizing these risks, you can make educated choices regarding the products you introduce to your home and the actions necessary to minimize their impact.

Recipe: DIY Non-Toxic Air Freshener

Ingredients:

1 cup distilled water

Ten drops of lavender essential oil

Five drops of eucalyptus essential oil.

Instructions:

Combine all ingredients in a spray bottle.

Shake well before use.

Spray lightly in rooms to freshen the air naturally.

Volatile Organic Compounds (VOCs): The Silent Pollutants

VOCs are chemicals that easily evaporate into the air, often undetectable by smell. They are a major contributor to poor indoor air quality. Found in a wide range of household items, such as paints, varnishes, furniture, carpets, and adhesives, VOCs can linger for months—or even years—after their initial application. Some of the most common VOCs include formaldehyde, benzene, and toluene. Each is associated with adverse health effects like respiratory irritation, headaches, and long-term risks, such as cancer.

Key Sources: Newly purchased furniture, freshly painted walls, and synthetic carpets.

Health Impacts: Prolonged exposure can lead to chronic respiratory issues, fatigue, and compromised immune function.

Synthetic Fragrances: A Hidden Chemical Cocktail

Synthetic fragrances in air fresheners, candles, detergents, and personal care products are another hidden danger. While they may create a pleasant aroma, they often contain a mix of harmful substances, including phthalates, a class of chemicals used to make fragrances last longer. Phthalates have been linked to hormone disruption, respiratory problems, and reproductive health issues.

Key Sources: Scented candles, plug-in air fresheners, laundry detergents, and perfumes.

Health Impacts: Frequent exposure to synthetic fragrances can contribute to headaches, asthma flare-ups, and endocrine disruption. They may also impact long-term reproductive and developmental health.

Cleaning Products: A Double-Edged Sword

While cleaning products are designed to remove dirt and germs, many conventional options contain harsh chemicals that can harm indoor air quality and skin health. Ingredients like ammonia, bleach, and quaternary ammonium compounds release fumes that can irritate the respiratory system and exacerbate allergies. Even "antibacterial" products may contain triclosan, a chemical linked to hormonal imbalance and bacterial resistance.

Key Sources: Multi-surface cleaners, dishwashing liquids, and disinfectants.

Health Impacts: Immediate effects include eye and throat irritation, while prolonged exposure can lead to chronic respiratory conditions and skin sensitivity.

Personal Care Products: Harm Lurking in Plain Sight

Many personal care items, such as shampoos, lotions, and makeup, contain potentially harmful ingredients such as parabens, sulfates, and synthetic dyes. These chemicals can be absorbed through the skin, contributing to hormonal imbalances and skin irritation.

Key Sources: Hair care products, skincare items, and cosmetics.

Health Impacts: Accumulated exposure may lead to hormonal disruption, allergic reactions, and an increased risk of certain cancers.

Steps to Mitigate Hidden Dangers

Identify and Replace Harmful Products

Start by reviewing the labels of items in your home. Look for certifications such as "organic," "non-toxic," or "low-VOC," which indicate safer alternatives. Replace conventional cleaning products with natural solutions like vinegar, baking soda, and essential oils. Personal care products are made with organic and plant-based ingredients.

Improve Ventilation

Ventilation is essential to reduce the concentration of harmful indoor air pollutants. Open windows regularly, use exhaust fans in kitchens and bathrooms and consider investing in a whole-house ventilation system.

Choose Natural Alternatives

For Fragrances: Replace synthetic air fresheners with essential oil diffusers or naturally scented soy candles.

For Cleaning: Use homemade cleaners made from natural ingredients, such as a mixture of vinegar and water for glass surfaces or baking soda for scrubbing.

For Furniture: Choose solid wood furniture with non-toxic finishes and avoid synthetic upholstery treated with flame retardants.

Prioritize Air Purification

Air purifiers with HEPA filters can remove a wide range of indoor pollutants, including VOCs, dust, and allergens. Houseplants like spider plants and peace lilies also contribute to cleaner air by naturally filtering toxins.

Be Cautious with New Purchases

When purchasing new items such as furniture, mattresses, or carpets, seek certifications like GreenGuard or OEKO-TEX. These indicate that the products have undergone testing for low chemical emissions. It's advisable to allow new products to "off-gas" outdoors or in a well-ventilated space before bringing them inside indoors.

Practice Minimalism

Having fewer items in your home can lead to a lower risk of hidden toxins. Embracing a minimalist decorating and furnishing style helps minimize clutter and limits unnecessary exposure to harmful substances and chemicals.

The Path to a Healthier Home

Identifying hidden hazards in everyday products is crucial for establishing a safer and healthier home. By pinpointing harmful chemicals like VOCs, phthalates, and synthetic fragrances and taking proactive steps to minimize or remove them, you create an environment that emphasizes health and wellness. Simple adjustments, such as opting for natural alternatives, enhancing airflow, and investing in air purification systems, can greatly improve your household and your family's quality of life. Keep in mind that the decisions you make today set the stage for a healthier, toxin-free tomorrow.

Chapter 6

Air Quality Matters

Air is essential to life, yet indoor air quality is often overlooked. Poor air quality can lead to respiratory issues, allergies, and chronic illnesses. This chapter delves into the factors that affect indoor air and how to address them effectively.

One of the first steps is identifying sources of indoor air pollution. These include smoke from cooking, off-gassing from new furniture, and the use of chemical-laden cleaning products. Awareness of these sources is crucial for implementing change.

Recipe: *Natural Air-Purifying Spray*

Ingredients:

1 cup distilled water

One tablespoon of witch hazel

Ten drops of peppermint essential oil.

Instructions:

Combine all ingredients in a spray bottle.

Shake well and spray in areas with stale air.

Enhancing ventilation is a straightforward yet effective way to improve air quality. By opening windows, utilizing exhaust fans, and installing air exchangers, you can increase fresh air circulation and lower the levels of indoor pollutants.

Houseplants serve more than just an aesthetic purpose; they function as natural air purifiers. Plants such as spider plants, snake plants, and peace lilies absorb toxins while releasing oxygen. This chapter will assist you in selecting and caring for the most effective air-purifying plants.

Controlling humidity levels is also essential. Excess humidity can foster mold and mildew, whereas low humidity can cause dry skin and respiratory issues. A dehumidifier or humidifier can help maintain a balanced environment.

We will also explore DIY air-purifying solutions, like natural sprays made from essential oils. These not only enhance air quality but also infuse your home with a pleasant, chemical-free aroma.

Lastly, monitoring air quality with modern devices, such as air quality sensors, can yield essential insights. By understanding your indoor air quality, you can implement targeted improvements to create a healthier home environment.

Chapter 7

Detoxifying Your Kitchen

The kitchen is the heart of the home, but it can also be a significant source of toxins. This chapter addresses common kitchen hazards from cookware to food storage and provides practical solutions.

Recipe: Natural Dish Soap

Ingredients:

One cup Castile soap

One tablespoon of baking soda

Ten drops of lemon essential oil.

Instructions:

Combine ingredients in a soap dispenser.

Shake well and use as needed for washing dishes.

While non-stick cookware is convenient, it often contains PFOAs, which release toxins at high temperatures. Transitioning to safer alternatives like stainless steel, cast iron, or ceramic is a worthwhile investment in your health.

Plastic food storage containers can leach harmful chemicals into your food, especially when heated. Glass or stainless-steel containers are safer for storing and reheating food.

Recipe: All-Purpose Counter Cleaner

Ingredients:

One cup distilled water

1/2 cup white vinegar

Ten drops of orange essential oil.

Instructions:

Mix all ingredients in a spray bottle.

Spray on counters and wipe with a cloth.

A key element of sustaining an off-grid lifestyle is the cleaning products we choose in the kitchen. Many commercial dish soaps, surface cleaners, and degreasers contain harsh chemicals that harm the environment and can leave residues impacting your health. These products often contribute to indoor air pollution and might pollute greywater systems, rendering them unsafe for garden reuse or in natural water cycles. In this chapter, you will discover simple and affordable recipes for non-toxic homemade alternatives. With just a few essential ingredients—like baking soda, vinegar, essential oils, and castile soap—you can create effective cleaners that are safe for both your family and the planet. These solutions are not only easy to prepare but also significantly decrease your dependence on plastic packaging, thereby reducing household waste.

Effective food storage is crucial in an off-grid kitchen, essential for reducing contamination and waste. Airtight containers form the backbone of any sustainable storage strategy. Durable and reusable options like glass jars, silicone bags, and stainless-steel containers keep food fresh and safe from pests. This chapter also explores natural preservation methods such as canning, fermenting, and dehydrating. Each technique is outlined with step-by-step instructions, including advice on sterilizing jars, creating the right fermentation environment, and selecting suitable foods for dehydration. These methods not only prolong the shelf life of your produce but also enable you to savor seasonal foods throughout the year without depending on a freezer electricity.

The significance of choosing organic and locally sourced produce. Conventional fruits and vegetables often undergo treatment with synthetic pesticides and fertilizers, which can negatively impact your health and the environment over time. By opting for organic alternatives and supporting local farmers, you minimize your exposure to harmful chemicals and encourage sustainable farming practices. This section offers practical guidance on safely washing and preparing fruits and vegetables. From basic rinsing methods to DIY vegetable washes using lemon juice or baking soda, these tips assist in removing residues and potential contaminants.

Lastly, detoxifying your kitchen involves more than just product and food selections; it encompasses your everyday habits. One of the most significant changes you can implement is reducing food waste. This chapter presents strategies like composting scraps, planning meals to prevent excess purchases, and innovative ways to use leftovers. Furthermore, incorporating reusable items like beeswax wraps, cloth napkins, and stainless-steel straws not only decreases waste but also supports a more self-sufficient way of living. Mindful consumption—the awareness of what you use and why—serves as a foundational principle for establishing a healthier, more sustainable kitchen atmosphere. Whether you choose to limit processed foods, cut back on single-use plastics, or simply value the resources involved in your meals, these practices foster a kitchen culture that nurtures both the planet and your well-being body.

Implementing the practical tips and solutions, you'll not only detoxify your kitchen but also transform it into a hub of health, sustainability, and mindful living.

Selecting Organic and Locally Sourced Produce

Selecting organic and locally sourced fruits and vegetables is an essential move towards establishing a healthier, more sustainable kitchen. Organic fruits and vegetables are cultivated without the use of synthetic pesticides, herbicides, or genetically modified organisms (GMOs), thereby decreasing your exposure to harmful chemicals. The gradual build-up of pesticide residues from conventional produce can adversely impact human health, potentially leading to issues like hormone disruption, neurological effects, and even certain types of cancer. Additionally, organic farming techniques enhance soil health, conserve water, and encourage biodiversity, making them a responsible choice for the environment choice.

Choosing locally sourced produce has many advantages. When you buy from local farmers, you minimize the carbon footprint linked to long-distance food transport, which in turn reduces greenhouse gas emissions and bolsters the local economy. Additionally, locally grown fruits and vegetables tend to be fresher and richer in nutrients since they are often picked at their peak ripeness and sold shortly after. Engaging with community-supported agriculture (CSA) programs and visiting farmers' markets are fantastic ways to obtain seasonal produce while establishing connections with the growers behind your food.

How to Wash and Prepare Fruits and Vegetables Properly

Regardless of whether you choose organic or locally sourced produce, it's crucial to wash and prepare it adequately to guarantee safety and enhance its nutritional benefits. Although organic farming reduces the use of harmful chemicals, natural contaminants such as soil, bacteria, or insects may still exist. Here are some effective steps to ensure your produce is clean and safe for consumption:

Rinse Thoroughly

Rinse produce under cool running water while gently rubbing its surface with your hands to eliminate dirt, bacteria, and handling residue. Refrain from using soap or detergent, as these should not be used food-safe.

Use Natural Cleaning Solutions

To tackle tougher residues, immerse fruits and vegetables in a homemade mixture of water, vinegar, and baking soda. A recommended ratio is 1 cup of vinegar to 4 cups of water, along with a teaspoon of baking soda for enhanced cleaning strength. Allow the produce to soak for 5 to 10 minutes, then rinse well. This technique works especially well for leafy greens, apples, and other items that have waxy surface crevices.

Peel When Necessary

Peeling thick-skinned produce like cucumbers, carrots, or potatoes can minimize exposure to leftover pesticides or contaminants. However, keep in mind that peels are often rich in nutrients, so consider peeling only when necessary necessary.

Dry Properly

Once washed, gently pat the produce dry with a clean towel or utilize a salad spinner for leafy greens. Adequate drying helps prevent spoilage due to moisture and prolongs the freshness of your produce.

5. *Store Thoughtfully*

To keep produce fresh, store washed items in breathable containers or wrap them in damp towels. It's important to separate different types of produce to prevent exposure to ethylene gas, which speeds up ripening spoilage.

Prioritize Certain Organic Choices

While purchasing entirely organic products is the best choice, it isn't always practical due to cost or availability. Instead, emphasize selecting organic options from the "Dirty Dozen" list—fruits and vegetables that are likely to have significant pesticide residues, including strawberries, spinach, kale, apples, and cherries. In contrast, items on the "Clean Fifteen" list, like avocados, pineapples, and sweet corn, are generally safer to buy conventionally since they have lower pesticide levels.

The Bigger Picture

Opting for organic and locally sourced produce goes beyond just steering clear of harmful chemicals; it's an investment in your health, a boost for sustainable farming, and a means to build a closer bond with your food. By diligently washing and preparing your produce, you ensure its safety while also elevating its flavor and nutritional benefits. This comprehensive philosophy toward food choice and preparation nurtures a kitchen environment that emphasizes health, sustainability, and conscious living.

Chapter 8

Water is Life: Ensuring a Safe and Sustainable Supply

WATER IS ESSENTIAL FOR life, yet its quality can differ greatly based on the source and treatment processes. Recognizing the significance of clean water and proactively ensuring a safe, sustainable supply is crucial for daily living and emergency readiness. This chapter examines the challenges related to water quality, investigates sustainable options, and provides practical solutions for making water safe for drinking, cooking, and other vital uses.

Recipe: DIY Fruit and Veggie Wash

Ingredients:

1 cup water

1 cup white vinegar

One tablespoon of baking soda

Instructions:

Mix ingredients in a large bowl.

Soak fruits and vegetables for 5 minutes.

Rinse thoroughly with clean water.

The Reality of Tap Water

Tap water is usually the easiest option for households, yet it often harbors contaminants that may threaten health. Common pollutants include:

Chlorine: Added to disinfect water, chlorine can leave an unpleasant taste and may react with organic matter to form harmful by-products.

Lead: Often leached from old plumbing systems, lead exposure can cause severe health issues, especially in children.

Microorganisms: While water treatment plants work to eliminate pathogens, tap water can still harbor bacteria, viruses, and parasites, particularly if the infrastructure is aging or damaged.

Improving Tap Water Quality

Investing in a reliable water filtration system can significantly enhance the quality of your tap water. Filtration options include:

Activated Carbon Filters: Effective at removing chlorine, sediment, and certain VOCs, improving taste and odor.

Reverse Osmosis Systems: These remove a wide range of contaminants, including lead, fluoride, and heavy metals.

Ultraviolet (UV) Purifiers: Useful for killing microorganisms without the need for chemical disinfectants.

The Hidden Costs of Bottled Water

While bottled water may seem like a convenient solution, it poses environmental and health concerns.

Environmental Impact: The production and disposal of plastic bottles contribute to pollution, with millions of tons of plastic waste ending up in oceans and landfills each year.

Health Risks: Chemicals like BPA (bisphenol A) and microplastics can leach into the water, particularly when bottles are exposed to heat or stored for long periods.

A Sustainable Alternative

Instead of relying on bottled water, consider filtering your tap water and using a reusable stainless steel or glass water bottle. This choice reduces waste and ensures access to cleaner, safer water.

Rainwater Harvesting: A Valuable Resource

Collecting rainwater is an excellent way to supplement your water supply for household and gardening purposes. However, it's essential to ensure its safety before using it.

Setting Up a Rainwater Collection System

1. ***Install Gutters and Downspouts***: These direct rainwater from your roof into a storage container or tank.

2. ***Choose a Storage Tank***: Opt for food-grade containers with secure lids to prevent contamination.

3. ***Use a First-Flush Diverter***: This device discards the initial flow of water, which may contain debris and pollutants from your roof.

4. ***Filter the Water***: Add a filtration system to remove sediment, leaves, and other impurities.

Safety Considerations

Regularly clean your collection system to prevent the growth of algae, bacteria, and mosquito breeding.

Treat rainwater with UV purification or boiling if you plan to use it for drinking or cooking.

Water for Cooking and Cleaning

The quality of water used in cooking and cleaning is often overlooked but can have significant health implications.

Washing Fruits and Vegetables: Rinsing produce with water may not be sufficient to remove pesticides and bacteria. Adding a splash of vinegar or baking soda to the water can enhance its effectiveness.

Cooking with Clean Water: Filtered or purified water prevents contaminants from leaching into food, improving its taste and safety.

DIY Water Purification Techniques

In emergency situations, access to clean water may become compromised. Having a few DIY purification methods at hand can be lifesaving:

Boiling: One of the simplest and most effective methods, boiling water for at least one minute kills bacteria, viruses, and parasites.

Activated Charcoal: This natural material can absorb impurities and improve water quality. It's particularly useful for removing unpleasant tastes and odors.

Solar Disinfection (SODIS): Placing water in clear plastic bottles and exposing them to direct sunlight for several hours can kill pathogens through UV radiation.

Bleach: In emergencies, unscented household bleach can disinfect water. Add 2 drops per liter of water, mix well, and let it sit for 30 minutes before drinking.

Maintaining Your Water Systems

Ensuring the safety of your water doesn't end with filtration or purification—it requires regular maintenance:

Replace Filters: Follow the manufacturer's guidelines for replacing filters in your water systems to maintain optimal performance.

Clean Storage Containers: Regularly sanitize tanks, bottles, and other water storage containers to prevent bacteria build-up.

Inspect Systems: Periodically check your rainwater harvesting setup or plumbing for leaks, cracks, or other issues.

Water's Role in a Sustainable Lifestyle

Clean water is essential not only for survival but also as a foundation for sustainable living. By learning about water sources, tackling contaminants, and adopting environmentally friendly methods such as rainwater harvesting and using reusable bottles, you can protect your water supply and minimize your ecological footprint. Whether for everyday needs or emergencies, the strategies discussed in this chapter will assist you in securing access to clean, safe water for both your family and community.

CHAPTER 9

GREEN CLEANING BASICS

Conventional cleaning products are filled with chemicals that can harm your health and the environment. Switching to green cleaning methods is not only better for you but also for the planet. This chapter introduces the basics of green cleaning and provides practical solutions.

Recipe: DIY All-Purpose Cleaner

Ingredients:

One cup distilled water

1/2 cup white vinegar

Ten drops tea tree essential oil

Ten drops of lemon essential oil.

Instructions:

Combine all ingredients in a spray bottle.

Shake well and use on surfaces like countertops, sinks, and tables.

Many commercial cleaners contain harsh chemicals, such as ammonia and chlorine, that can irritate the skin and lungs. However, natural ingredients like vinegar, baking soda, and essential oils can create effective cleaners without toxic side effects.

Recipe: Natural Glass Cleaner

Ingredients:

One cup distilled water

One cup rubbing alcohol.

One tablespoon of white vinegar

Instructions:

Mix all ingredients in a spray bottle.

Spray on glass surfaces and wipe with a lint-free cloth.

Many commercial cleaners contain harsh chemicals, such as ammonia and chlorine, that can irritate the skin and lungs. In contrast, natural ingredients such as vinegar, baking soda, and essential oils can create effective cleaning solutions without toxic side effects.

Homemade all-purpose cleaners are versatile and simple to create. A basic combination of vinegar, water, and a few drops of essential oil can effectively clean most surfaces in your home. This chapter provides recipes and helpful tips for making these solutions.

Natural disinfectants, such as hydrogen peroxide, alcohol, and essential oils such as tea tree or eucalyptus, are also crucial in green cleaning. These disinfectants offer safe and effective antimicrobial properties. This section teaches you how to create and use them in your home.

Green cleaning goes beyond cleaning solutions **and** includes the tools you use. Microfiber cloths, reusable mop pads, and biodegradable sponges are eco-friendly alternatives to conventional cleaning supplies. Choosing these tools decreases waste and encourages sustainability.

Moreover, knowing the proper techniques for green cleaning enhances effectiveness. For instance, giving natural disinfectants a few minutes to sit improves their germ-killing capabilities. This chapter also presents troubleshooting advice for common cleaning issues.

Green cleaning is more than just a health choice; it's a lifestyle commitment that reflects environmental responsibility. By adopting these practices, you contribute to a healthier home and a cleaner planet.

Chapter 10

Revamping Your Laundry Routine

Laundry plays a crucial role in our daily routine, but traditional laundry products often bring harmful chemicals into our homes and the environment. Numerous detergents and fabric softeners include synthetic fragrances, dyes, and optical brighteners, which can lead to skin irritation and allergies.

Recipe: DIY Laundry Detergent

Ingredients:

One cup washing soda.

One cup baking soda

1/2 cup grated Castile soap

Instructions:

Mix all ingredients in an airtight container.

Use two tablespoons per load for a standard washer and one tablespoon for HE washers.

Switching to eco-friendly laundry detergents or making your own is an excellent first step. You can create an effective detergent by mixing washing soda, baking soda, and castile soap. This detergent is gentle on clothes and the environment. Adding white vinegar during the rinse cycle serves as a natural fabric softener.

Another concern is dryer sheets, which often contain chemicals that leave residue on clothes. Instead, wool dryer balls make a fantastic alternative. You can enhance their scent by infusing them with essential oils. Additionally, these balls help reduce drying time, leading to energy savings.

It's also vital to understand your washing machine's impact. Front-loading machines are typically more energy-efficient and consume less water. Regular maintenance, including cleaning the drum and using a descaler, ensures optimal performance and helps prevent mold build-up.

You can substitute commercial stain removers with natural alternatives. A paste made of baking soda and water, or a mixture of hydrogen peroxide and liquid soap can effectively handle most stains without harsh chemicals. Pre-soaking clothes in these solutions can enhance their stain-removing power.

Tip: Natural Stain Remover

Ingredients:

1/4 cup hydrogen peroxide

1/4 cup baking soda

One tablespoon Castile soap

Instructions:

Mix into a paste.

Apply to stains and let sit for 15 minutes before washing.

Lastly, consider how your laundry habits affect the environment. Washing clothes in cold water, air drying when possible, and using biodegradable products help lessen your carbon footprint. Improving your laundry practices can safeguard your family's health while promoting a healthier planet.

Chapter 11

Non-Toxic Bedroom Bliss

The bedroom ought to be a relaxing sanctuary, but it frequently harbors hidden toxins. Elements like mattresses, bedding, and furniture can all contribute to indoor air pollution, impacting your health.

Recipe: Linen Spray for Restful Sleep

Ingredients:

One cup distilled water

Two tablespoons vodka or witch hazel

Ten drops of lavender essential oil

Five drops of chamomile essential oil.

Instructions:

Mix all ingredients in a spray bottle.

Lightly mist linens before bed.

Many standard mattresses use polyurethane foam and flame retardants. Instead, choose organic mattresses made from natural materials like latex, wool, and cotton. These alternatives are free of harmful chemicals and offer excellent support and comfort.

Bedding is another critical consideration. Synthetic fabrics may contain dyes and chemical treatments that can irritate sensitive skin. Organic cotton, bamboo, and linen serve as great breathable and hypoallergenic options. Washing new bedding with a natural detergent before use can further minimize chemical exposure.

Furniture and flooring materials can also release VOCs. Solid wood furniture finished with non-toxic products and natural fiber rugs are safer choices. Avoid synthetic carpets, which can harbor allergens and emit harmful chemicals over time.

Creating a sleep-friendly environment entails more than just selecting appropriate materials. Limiting electronic devices and using blackout curtains can enhance sleep quality. Introducing air-purifying plants like lavender or jasmine provides a soothing ambiance while improving air quality.

Aromatherapy can help create a toxin-free bedroom. Diffusing essential oils such as lavender or chamomile fosters relaxation and sleep. By addressing these factors, you can transform your bedroom into a true sanctuary for health and well-being tranquility.

Chapter 12

Living Room Liberation

The living room is often the central gathering place in a home but can also harbor toxins. Upholstery, carpets, and electronic devices contribute to poor indoor air quality and health risks.

Recipe: DIY Fabric Freshener

Ingredients:

One cup distilled water

One tablespoon of baking soda

Ten drops of lavender essential oil.

Instructions:

Combine ingredients in a spray bottle.

Lightly mist upholstery and carpets to freshen.

Furniture made from synthetic fabrics and foam typically includes flame retardants and formaldehyde. Opting for furniture crafted from natural materials like wool, cotton, or leather can significantly decrease exposure to these harmful substances. Furthermore, seeking certifications such as GREENGUARD or OEKO-TEX can offer additional reassurance.

Carpets and rugs tend to trap allergens, dust, and chemicals. If replacing the carpet isn't feasible, regular vacuuming with a HEPA filter and steam cleaning can help mitigate these risks. Natural fiber rugs, such as jute or sisal, serve as excellent alternatives to their synthetic counterparts.

Electronic devices produce electromagnetic fields (EMFs) and can harbor dust, especially those containing flame retardants. Reducing electronics in the living room and maintaining cleanliness can effectively lessen exposure. Additionally, arranging furniture to promote enhanced airflow and incorporating air-purifying plants further improve the surrounding environment.

Air fresheners and candles are common sources of synthetic fragrances. Substituting these with essential oil diffusers or beeswax candles offers a natural alternative that enriches the atmosphere without introducing harmful chemicals.

Decluttering the living room can significantly benefit mental health. Adopting a minimalist approach helps lower stress levels and reduces the build-up of dust and allergens. By clearing your living room, you create a space that promotes health and connection to toxins.

Chapter 13

Bathroom Detox

The bathroom is one of the most toxic areas in the home due to the vast array of personal care and cleaning products used daily. Many of these items contain synthetic fragrances, parabens, and phthalates, which can disrupt hormones and irritate the skin.

Recipe: Non-Toxic Bathroom Cleaner

Ingredients:

One cup white vinegar

One cup distilled water

Ten drops tea tree essential oil

Ten drops of lemon essential oil.

Instructions:

Mix all ingredients in a spray bottle.

Spray surfaces and let sit for a few minutes.

Wipe clean with a cloth or sponge.

Switching to natural personal care products is an effective way to reduce chemical exposure. Look for items made with organic ingredients and free from synthetic additives. DIY toothpaste, deodorant, and body wash recipes can be customized to suit your preferences and skin type.

Recipe: DIY Natural Toothpaste

Ingredients:

Two tablespoons of coconut oil

One tablespoon of baking soda

Five drops of peppermint essential oil.

Instructions:

Mix ingredients into a paste.

Store in a small jar and use a pea-sized amount for brushing.

PVC shower curtains emit harmful chemicals over time. Instead, choose fabric or PEVA options that are safer and more sustainable. Regular cleaning of the shower with vinegar and baking soda helps prevent mold growth and reduces the need for harsh chemicals.

Toiletries like toilet paper and sanitary items frequently contain bleaches and dyes. Opting for unbleached, organic alternatives can lower exposure to these substances. Furthermore, using a bidet attachment can decrease reliance on disposable products.

Water conservation is also crucial for bathroom detox. Installing low-flow fixtures and repairing leaks can reduce water waste and lower utility costs. Reusing greywater for outdoor purposes is an excellent way to manage resources responsibly.

Lastly, incorporating plants into your bathroom can enhance air quality and create a spa-like ambiance. Plants such as aloe vera and ferns thrive in humid conditions and assist in air purification. A detoxed bathroom supports health, sustainability, and wellbeing relaxation.

Chapter 14

Decluttering for Health

Clutter influences more than the appearance of your home; it can also affect your mental and physical health. A messy environment often contains dust, allergens, and stress, which makes decluttering an essential aspect of maintaining your home detoxification.

Recipe: DIY Natural Dusting Spray

Ingredients:

One cup distilled water

1/4 cup white vinegar

One tablespoon of olive oil

Ten drops of lemon essential oil.

Instructions:

Combine ingredients in a spray bottle.

Shake well before each use.

Spray onto surfaces and wipe with a microfiber cloth.

Begin by sorting your items into three categories: keep, donate, and discard. This organized method streamlines the process and directs attention to items that truly enrich your life. Storage solutions like bins and baskets help maintain the organization and accessibility of the items you choose to keep.

Equally important is digital decluttering. Reducing electronic waste by responsibly recycling old devices and organizing your digital files alleviates stress and enhances productivity. A tidy digital space complements a physically clutter-free environment.

Additionally, it is vital to reassess your sentimental items. While it's crucial to cherish memories, limiting keepsakes to a select few meaningful pieces helps avoid clutter. Consider using digital photo albums or shadow boxes to showcase precious memories without contributing to physical disarray.

The advantages of decluttering reach beyond your home. Donating items you no longer use to local charities promotes sustainability and supports those in need. Selling valuable items online can also generate extra income while minimizing waste.

Keeping your home clutter-free necessitates consistent habits. Allocating time each month to assess and organize your belongings ensures ongoing success. By adopting minimalism, you cultivate a living space that is both tidy, soothing, and functional.

Chapter 15

Safe Flooring Solutions

Your home's flooring choices greatly affect indoor air quality and your overall health. Numerous common flooring options, including vinyl and synthetic carpets, are known to contain toxic substances such as phthalates, formaldehyde, and VOCs. This chapter aims to highlight safer alternatives and promote healthier options floors.

Recipe: DIY Floor Cleaner

Ingredients:

One gallon warm water

1/4 cup Castile soap

Ten drops of eucalyptus essential oil.

Instructions:

Mix all ingredients in a bucket.

Use a mop or cloth to clean floors as needed.

Hardwood floors are valued for their strength and natural appearance. To minimize VOC emissions, select sustainably sourced options with non-toxic finishes. Engineered wood featuring low-VOC adhesives presents a viable alternative.

Bamboo and cork are eco-friendly, renewable, and stylish flooring solutions. They also resist mold and mildew, making them suitable for humid areas. However, ensure that the adhesives used in their installation are free of formaldehyde.

While carpets provide comfort, they can collect allergens, dust, and harmful chemicals. If you prefer carpet, go for natural fiber options like wool, jute, or sisal. These materials are biodegradable and devoid of synthetic dyes and treatments. Regular vacuuming with a HEPA filter, along with steam cleaning, can further minimize allergens.

Tile and stone floors are also excellent choices for durability and ease of cleaning. To lessen environmental impact, seek tiles made from natural clay or recycled materials. Avoid using synthetic sealants, opting instead for water-based or low-VOC alternatives.

Proper maintenance is essential for safe flooring. Utilizing natural cleaning solutions, such as vinegar and water mixture, helps care for your floors without introducing harmful toxins. Following these suggestions fosters a healthier foundation home.

Chapter 16

Healthy Walls and Paints

The home's walls play a bigger role in indoor air quality than you might realize. Traditional paints and wall treatments frequently emit VOCs, which can affect your well-being long after they've been applied. This chapter investigates healthier alternatives for wall coverings and paints.

Recipe: DIY Natural Wall Cleaner

Ingredients:

One gallon warm water

1/2 cup white vinegar

1/4 cup baking soda

Instructions:

Mix all ingredients in a bucket.

Use a sponge or cloth to clean the walls, then rinse with clean water.

Low-VOC and zero-VOC paints are readily available and significantly reduce indoor air toxicity. These options perform similarly to traditional paints while being safer for your family and the environment. Always verify labels for certifications to guarantee that the product complies with safety requirements.

Another option is natural paints crafted from clay, milk, or plant-based oils. These paints contain no synthetic chemicals and provide a distinctive appearance. They are particularly beneficial for those with chemical sensitivities.

Wallpaper that includes vinyl or is applied with adhesives that release VOCs may also contribute to toxic exposure. To minimize this risk, choose wallpaper made from natural fibers and use water-based adhesives. It's also important to ensure proper ventilation during installation.

Make thoughtful choices when selecting wall finishes, such as plasters and sealants. Lime or clay plasters are natural alternatives that enhance texture and depth and promote better indoor air quality. Avoid synthetic finishes, which can emit harmful chemicals.

Regular wall maintenance is also crucial. Cleaning with natural solutions can help prevent mold and mildew growth, and promptly addressing any water damage is essential for preventing structural issues and health risks.

Focussing on healthy wall treatments can create a visually pleasing environment that supports well-being. The right selections can transform your walls into a protective barrier against hazards and toxins.

Chapter 17

The Role of Plants in Detoxification

Houseplants are not only decorative elements but also powerful allies for enhancing indoor air quality. This chapter explores their advantages and offers guidance on how to integrate them effectively into your home.

Recipe: DIY Natural Fertilizer for Houseplants

Ingredients:

One banana peel

One tablespoon used coffee grounds.

One liter water

Instructions:

Blend all ingredients until smooth.

Use the mixture as a natural fertilizer for your houseplants.

Snake plants, spider plants, and peace lilies effectively filter common indoor pollutants, including benzene, formaldehyde, and carbon monoxide. They require minimal care and flourish in various conditions, making them perfect for any household.

For those seeking better sleep, lavender and jasmine emit soothing fragrances that aid relaxation. Positioning these plants in the bedroom can improve sleep quality and alleviate stress.

Proper placement of plants is crucial for their purifying abilities. Clustering plants in poorly ventilated areas, like corners or near electronic devices, can enhance air purification. Periodically rotating them ensures they receive adequate light exposure and helps maintain their health.

Installing a living wall or vertical garden is a smart, space-efficient way to add greenery to your home. These setups enhance air quality and add a stunning visual touch to your environment. For optimal results, select plants suitable for your specific climate and indoor conditions.

Routine care is essential for houseplants' longevity and efficacy. Regular watering, pruning, and feeding with organic fertilizers keep them thriving. Watching for pests and applying natural remedies guarantees a non-toxic approach.

Integrating plants into your living space is a straightforward yet powerful method of purifying your surroundings. In addition to their air-cleaning capabilities, they infuse vitality and foster a connection to nature, enriching your physical and emotional well-being.

Chapter 18

Kitchen Pantry Detox

The kitchen pantry is the heart of your kitchen, but it may also harbor hidden toxins. Processed foods, plastic packaging, and synthetic additives pose health risks. This chapter emphasizes the importance of establishing a toxin-free pantry.

Recipe: DIY Pantry Deodorizer

Ingredients:

1/2 cup baking soda

Ten drops of grapefruit essential oil.

Instructions:

Mix ingredients and place in an open jar.

Store the jar in your pantry to absorb odors naturally.

Assess the items in your pantry. Eliminate products containing artificial colors, flavors, and preservatives. Prioritize whole, unprocessed foods that offer nutritional benefits without harmful additives.

Storage solutions are crucial for preserving a healthy pantry. Swap plastic containers for glass jars or stainless-steel alternatives. These materials are nonreactive and help keep food fresh longer. Additionally, airtight containers help prevent pest infestations.

Think about the effects of pesticides on conventionally farmed produce. Opt for organic **choices,** when possible, to lessen your exposure. Purchasing in bulk from reliable sources reduces packaging waste and guarantees quality for dry goods like grains and legumes.

Spices and herbs, often neglected, can harbor hidden toxins if not stored appropriately. To prevent contamination, store them in cool, dark environments and select organic options. Making your spice blends is a fun and healthful alternative.

Organizing your pantry enhances its efficiency and promotes healthier choices. Arrange items by category and label containers for easy access. A well-organized pantry diminishes the likelihood of reaching for processed snacks.

Detoxifying your kitchen pantry lays the groundwork for healthier cooking and eating habits. This small yet impactful adjustment can significantly influence your overall well-being lifestyle.

Chapter 19

Outdoor Spaces for Health

Creating toxin-free outdoor spaces is just as crucial as detoxifying your home's interior. Outdoor environments often harbor chemical-laden fertilizers, pesticides, and polluted air, all of which can affect health. This chapter delves into how to turn your outdoor area into a wellness sanctuary.

Start with soil health, the core of a flourishing garden. Evaluate your soil for toxins and detoxify it if needed, using organic compost and natural soil amendments. Embrace organic gardening methods to nurture a vibrant, chemical-free landscape. Experiment with this recipe for natural fertilizer.

Recipe: Natural Fertilizer

Ingredients:

One part compost

One part aged manure

One part organic bone meal

Instructions:

Combine all ingredients and mix thoroughly.

Spread evenly over your garden beds and work into the soil.

Pesticides and herbicides are common culprits in outdoor pollution. Replace these with natural alternatives such as neem oil, diatomaceous earth, or companion planting to repel pests and weeds without harming beneficial organisms. Try this natural pest-repellent spray:

Recipe: Natural Pest Spray

Ingredients:

Two cups water

Two teaspoons of neem oil

One teaspoon liquid Castile soap

Instructions:

Combine all ingredients in a spray bottle.

Shake well and spray directly on plants.

Water features such as ponds and fountains enhance outdoor beauty and air quality. It's important to keep them clean with natural cleaners and to utilize aquatic plants for filtering and oxygenating the water.

Seating and play areas should be free from harmful materials. Choose outdoor furniture made from untreated wood, recycled products, or non-toxic stains. For children, design play areas using natural materials like sand or bark mulch.

In addition, planting native plants helps lower water usage and increases biodiversity. Trees and shrubs provide shade and serve as natural air purifiers, minimizing dust and pollutants in your outdoor environment.

Creating a toxin-free outdoor area extends your home's sanctuary, providing a peaceful spot for relaxation, play, and connection to nature. Ensuring these spaces are chemical-free is just as crucial as detoxifying your indoors. Outdoor areas often harbor chemical-filled fertilizers, pesticides, and polluted air, all of which can negatively affect health. This chapter discusses transforming your outdoor.

Chapter 20

Smart Technology Choices

Technology plays a crucial role in our daily lives, but it also introduces electromagnetic fields (EMFs) and other risks into our environments. This chapter discusses ways to integrate technology wisely to create a safer and healthier home.

The first step is to understand EMFs. As scientific knowledge develops, it's generally wise to minimize exposure. Consider switching off Wi-Fi routers during the night, opting for wired connections when feasible, and keeping devices like laptops and smartphones at a distance when in use.

While smart home devices offer convenience, they can contribute to technology overload. Opt for products that emphasize energy efficiency and low emissions. Many brands now provide eco-friendly alternatives with a lower environmental footprint. You can also use applications to monitor your device usage and electricity consumption to improve management.

If privacy and data security are important to you, choose devices with strong encryption and limit data sharing. This will safeguard your personal information and lower the risk of unnecessary technology exposure.

Lighting significantly affects health, and smart lighting systems can replicate natural light cycles. Using dimmable, color-adjustable LED lights can help regulate circadian rhythms, enhancing sleep quality and overall health. Implement a smart lighting app to manage brightness changes throughout the day.

Establish technology usage boundaries, such as creating areas without devices or setting specific charging zones. This promotes a healthier equilibrium between digital interaction and physical presence.

With careful technology selections, you can reap the rewards of modern.

Tech Detox Checklist

Turn off Wi-Fi at night.

Reduce EMF exposure by keeping devices at a distance.

Set device-free zones (e.g., bedrooms, dining areas).

Use apps to monitor and limit screen time.

Opt for low-energy smart devices with privacy features. Technology is integral to modern life, but it also introduces electromagnetic fields (EMFs) and other risks into our living spaces. This chapter addresses how to integrate technology wisely for a safer and healthier home.

Understanding EMFs is the first step. While the science is still evolving, minimizing exposure is generally considered a prudent approach. To this end, turn off Wi-Fi routers at night, use wired connections where possible, and place devices like laptops and cell phones away from your body when in use.

Though convenient, smart home devices can add to the tech clutter. Choose products that prioritize energy efficiency and low emissions. Many brands now offer eco-friendly options with reduced environmental impact.

For those concerned about privacy and data security, select devices with robust encryption and minimal data sharing. This not only protects personal information but also reduces the potential for unnecessary tech exposure.

Lighting plays a crucial role in health, and smart lighting systems can mimic natural light cycles. Dimmable, color-changing LED lights help regulate circadian rhythms, improving sleep and overall well-being.

Set boundaries for technology usage, such as creating device-free zones or designated charging areas. This encourages a healthier balance between digital engagement and physical presence.

By making thoughtful technology choices, you can enjoy the benefits of modern conveniences while minimizing their potential downsides.

Chapter 21

The Impact of Light and Sound

Light and sound are essential components of a healthy living environment. Poor lighting and excessive noise can negatively affect sleep, mood, and productivity. This chapter explores ways to optimize light and sound for a harmonious home.

Natural light is the best source of illumination. Maximizing sunlight by using sheer curtains, strategically placed mirrors, and arranging furniture to avoid blocking Skylights and light tubes can introduce more daylight into dimming room areas. For artificial lighting, prioritize LED bulbs with adjustable color temperatures. Warm light is ideal for evenings, while cool light boosts focus during the day. Install dimmers to control brightness and create a soothing ambiance.

Soundproofing techniques can help reduce noise pollution. Thick curtains, rugs, and acoustic panels absorb sound and create a quieter environment. Double-glazed windows are another effective option for blocking external noise. Try this DIY acoustic panel recipe:

Recipe: DIY Acoustic Panels

Materials:

Plywood (cut to size)

Acoustic foam panels

Fabric (to cover the panel)

Spray adhesive

Instructions:

Attach the acoustic foam to the plywood using spray adhesive.

Cover the panel with fabric and staple it securely at the back.

Mount the panel on walls where soundproofing is needed.

White noise machines or natural soundscapes can mask disruptive sounds and promote relaxation. These are particularly useful in bedrooms or workspaces.

Music and sound therapy are powerful tools for mental and emotional health. Playing calming music or nature sounds can enhance mood and concentration. Consider adding smart speakers to integrate soundscapes seamlessly into your daily routine.

Balancing light and sound creates an environment that nurtures both body and mind, contributing to overall well-being. Light and sound are essential components of a healthy living environment. Poor lighting and excessive noise can negatively affect sleep, mood, and productivity. This chapter explores ways to optimize light and sound for a harmonious home.

Natural light is the best source of illumination. Maximize sunlight by using sheer curtains, strategically placing mirrors, and arranging furniture to avoid blocking windows. Skylights or light tubes can bring additional daylight into darker areas.

For artificial lighting, prioritize LED bulbs with adjustable color temperatures. Warm light is ideal for evenings, while cool light boosts focus during the day. Install dimmers to control brightness and create a soothing ambiance.

Soundproofing techniques can help reduce noise pollution. Thick curtains, rugs, and acoustic panels absorb sound and create a quieter environment. Double-glazed windows are another effective option for blocking external noise.

White noise machines or nature soundscapes can mask disruptive sounds and promote relaxation. These are particularly useful in bedrooms or workspaces.

Music and sound therapy are powerful tools for mental and emotional health. Playing calming music or nature sounds can enhance mood and concentration. Consider adding smart speakers to integrate soundscapes seamlessly into your daily routine.

Balancing light and sound, you create an environment that nurtures both body and mind, contributing to overall well-being.

Chapter 22

Seasonal Detox Strategies

Every season presents distinct challenges and opportunities for detoxifying your home. This chapter offers specific strategies to maintain a toxin-free environment throughout the year.

Spring is ideal for thorough cleaning. Open windows to enhance airflow, clean air vents, and change filters. Utilize natural cleaning agents such as vinegar and baking soda to remove winter dirt. Consider this spring-cleaning approach recipe:

Recipe: Spring Cleaning Spray

Ingredients:

One cup white vinegar

One cup water

Ten drops of lemon essential oil

Instructions:

Mix all ingredients in a spray bottle.

Use on surfaces like countertops, sinks, and tables.

Wipe clean with a microfiber cloth.

Summer requires controlling humidity. Excess moisture can promote mold growth, so utilize dehumidifiers and promptly repair leaks. Natural pest deterrents like citronella and essential oils effectively ward off insects. Consider using this natural bug repellent:

Recipe: Bug Repellent Spray

Ingredients:

One cup witch hazel

ten drops citronella essential oil

10 drops tea tree essential oil

Instructions:

Combine ingredients in a spray bottle.

Shake well before each use.

Spray around doorways, windows, and outdoor seating areas.

Autumn is perfect for readying your home for the colder months. Check and seal your windows and doors to block drafts and minimize energy loss. Replace synthetic air fresheners with natural alternatives such as cinnamon and cloves to foster a warm ambiance. Prepare this stovetop potpourri:

Recipe: Cozy Autumn Potpourri

Ingredients:

One orange, sliced

Two cinnamon sticks

Four cloves

Two cups water

Instructions:

Add all ingredients to a small pot.

Simmer on low heat, adding water as needed.

Enjoy the natural aroma throughout your home.

Winter requires careful attention to indoor air quality. Use humidifiers to combat dry air and add houseplants to enhance oxygen levels. Wash and store heavy fabrics like curtains and blankets to prevent dust accumulation. Try this plant care tip for winter:

Tip: Winter Plant Care

Group plants together to maintain humidity.

Avoid overwatering as plants grow slower in winter.

Wipe leaves with a damp cloth to keep them dust-free.

Seasonal detox involves adopting good habits. Regularly rotate pantry staples to maintain freshness and declutter your wardrobes to accommodate seasonal clothing. Consistent small efforts ensure your home remains healthy and welcoming year-round. Each season introduces its own challenges and opportunities for refreshing your living space. This chapter offers customized strategies to maintain a toxin-free home throughout the year.

Spring is the ideal time for a thorough cleaning. Open windows for better ventilation, clean your air vents, and replace filters. To remove winter dirt, use natural cleaners like vinegar and baking soda.

In summer, managing humidity is crucial. High humidity can promote mold growth, so employ dehumidifiers and promptly repair any leaks. Natural pest deterrents, such as citronella and essential oils, help keep insects away.

Autumn is the perfect season to prepare your home for the colder months. Check and seal windows and doors to block drafts and prevent energy loss. Replace synthetic air fresheners with natural alternatives like cinnamon and cloves to create a warm atmosphere.

In winter, focus on improving indoor air quality. Use humidifiers to combat dry air and incorporate houseplants to increase oxygen levels. Clean and store heavy fabrics like curtains and blankets to avoid dust build-up.

Seasonal detox also emphasizes developing habits. Rotate pantry items for freshness and clear out wardrobes for seasonal clothing. Consistent small actions keep your home healthy and welcoming throughout the year.

Chapter 23

Building a Non-Toxic Community

Detoxifying your home is merely the first step; sharing insights and cultivating a supportive community enhances the effect. This chapter delves into how to nurture connections and promote collective action.

Begin by organizing workshops or informational gatherings in your community. Subjects such as DIY cleaning methods, organic gardening, or toxin-free baby care may draw interest and motivate others to act. Consider using this straightforward DIY recipe as part of a workshop starter:

Recipe: DIY All-Purpose Cleaner

Ingredients:

Two cups distilled water.

Two tablespoons castile soap

Ten drops lavender essential oil

Instructions:

Mix all ingredients in a spray bottle.

Demonstrate its use on various surfaces during your workshop.

Social media platforms are effective tools for raising awareness. Establish groups or pages to disseminate tips, success stories, and helpful resources. Eye-catching visuals and before-and-after pictures can inspire others to join the cause. When sharing posts, use hashtags such as #ToxinFreeLiving or #CleanGreenCommunity.

Partner with local businesses to highlight eco-friendly products and practices. Supporting farmers' markets, green stores, and sustainable brands bolsters the community's commitment to health and environmental sustainability. Collaborate with these entities to organize events or provide discounts.

Advocate for policy changes that promote toxin-free living by campaigning for the prohibition of harmful chemicals or encouraging schools and workplaces to implement healthier practices. Offer templates for petitions and sample letters to assist others in getting involved.

Honor milestones and successes by organizing community gatherings like clean-up events, plant exchanges, or sustainability fairs. Acknowledging shared accomplishments cultivates a sense of pride and dedication.

Creating a non-toxic community, you initiate a ripple effect that reaches well beyond your home, aiding in the creation of a healthier planet. Detoxifying your living space is merely the first step; sharing knowledge and fostering a supportive community amplifies the overall impact. This chapter discusses strategies for building connections and encouraging collaborative efforts.

Organizing workshops or informational sessions within your community. Topics such as DIY cleaning solutions, organic gardening, or toxin-free baby care can draw interest and motivate others to make positive changes. Social media platforms are powerful tools for raising awareness. Establish groups or pages to share tips, success stories, and resources. Eye-catching visuals and before-and-after photos can inspire others to join the cause

Partner with local businesses to highlight eco-friendly products and practices. Support farmers' markets, green stores, and sustainable brands to bolster the community's commitment to health and sustainability. Advocate for policy changes that foster toxin-free living by campaigning to prohibit harmful chemicals or encourage healthier practices in schools and workplaces.

Celebrate milestones and successes by organizing community gatherings like clean-up events, plant exchanges, or sustainability fairs. Acknowledging shared accomplishments cultivates a sense of pride and dedication.

A non-toxic community creates a ripple effect that extends well beyond your home, contributing to a healthier future planet.

Chapter 24

Sustaining Your Toxin-Free Lifestyle

A toxin-free lifestyle is a journey, not a destination. This chapter provides strategies for maintaining the changes you've made and growing in your commitment to health and sustainability.

Create a maintenance schedule to stay on track. Regularly inspect your home for new sources of toxins and update your practices as needed. Seasonal checklists can help you stay organized. Use this sample checklist:

Sample Maintenance Checklist

Inspect air filters and replace them if needed.

Check for mold in damp areas.

Rotate pantry staples and check expiration dates.

Wash and refresh reusable items like cloth bags and cleaning rags.

Stay updated on the latest trends and research in toxin-free living. You can remain engaged and inspired by subscribing to newsletters, attending webinars, and becoming part of online communities. Share reliable resources like eco-friendly blogs and online forums.

Engage your family in building a toxin-free home. To encourage collaboration, assign roles like watering plants, sorting recycling, or preparing DIY cleaners. Teaching children about sustainability instills enduring habits. Use games or challenges to make the learning process fun.

Investigate new avenues for detoxification. This could mean switching to eco-friendly transportation, supporting sustainable fashion, or minimizing waste through composting and minimalism. Check out this beginner's guide to composting tip:

Tip: Easy Composting at Home

Start with a small bin or pile.

Add food scraps (vegetables, fruits) and yard waste.

Avoid dairy, meat, or greasy items to prevent odors.

Turn regularly to speed up decomposition.

Celebrate your progress and share your journey. Reflect on how far you've come and set new goals to deepen your impact. Sharing your story can inspire others and reinforce your commitment. Host "progress parties" to review achievements with family and friends.

Sustaining a toxin-free lifestyle is about consistency and growth. By embracing it as an ongoing process, you ensure a healthier future for yourself, your loved ones, and the planet. A toxin-free lifestyle is a journey, not a destination. This chapter provides strategies for maintaining the changes you've made and continuing to grow in your commitment to health and sustainability.

Create a maintenance schedule to stay on track. Inspect your home regularly for new sources of toxins and update your practices as needed. Seasonal checklists can help you stay organized.

Stay informed about emerging trends and research in toxin-free living by subscribing to newsletters, attending webinars, and joining online communities. These activities will keep you engaged and motivated.

Involve your family in maintaining a toxin-free home. Assign tasks like watering plants, sorting recycling, or mixing DIY cleaners to make it a collaborative effort. Teaching children about sustainability instills lifelong habits.

Explore new areas of detoxification. This might include transitioning to eco-friendly transportation, supporting sustainable fashion, or reducing waste through composting and minimalism.

Celebrate your progress and share your journey. Reflect on how far you've come and set new goals to deepen your impact. Sharing your story can inspire others and reinforce your commitment.

Sustaining a toxin-free lifestyle is about consistency and growth. By embracing it as an ongoing process, you ensure a healthier future for yourself, your loved ones, and the planet.

Chapter 25

Recipes for the Home: Cleaning Solutions

These recipes provide an eco-friendly and holistic approach to cleaning, personal care, and wellness

Natural Pine Needle All-Purpose Cleaner

Ingredients:

One cup fresh pine needles (chopped for better extraction)

Two cups white vinegar

One cup distilled water

One tablespoon baking soda (optional)

Ten drops pine essential oil (optional)

A glass spray bottle

Instructions:

Prepare the Pine Needles:

Rinse fresh pine needles to remove dirt.

Chop into small pieces to release natural oils.

Infuse the Vinegar:

Place chopped pine needles into a clean glass jar.

Cover with vinegar and seal the jar tightly.

Let sit in a cool, dark place for 2 weeks. Shake occasionally.

Strain the Infusion:

Strain the vinegar to remove pine needles.

Mix the Cleaner:

Combine 1 cup infused vinegar, 1 cup distilled water, and optional ingredients (baking soda, pine essential oil) in a spray bottle.

Shake Before Use:

Shake the bottle before each use.

All-Purpose Cleaner

Ingredients:

One cup distilled water

One cup white vinegar

Ten drops essential oil (lemon, lavender, or tea tree)

One tablespoon baking soda (optional)

Instructions:

    1. Combine all ingredients in a spray bottle.

    2. Shake well before each use.

    3. Use on countertops, glass, and most hard surfaces.

Glass and Mirror Cleaner

Ingredients:

One cup distilled water

One cup white vinegar

One teaspoon cornstarch

Instructions:

    1. Mix ingredients in a spray bottle.

2. Shake well.

3. Spray onto glass or mirrors and wipe clean with a microfiber cloth.

Non-Toxic Floor Cleaner

Ingredients:

One gallon warm water

1/2 cup white vinegar

2-3 drops dish soap

Five drops essential oil (eucalyptus or lemon)

Instructions:

1. Mix ingredients in a mop bucket.

2. Mop floors as usual, avoiding excessive water on wood surfaces.

Natural Bathroom Scrub

Ingredients:

1/2 cup baking soda

1/4 cup liquid castile soap

One tablespoon hydrogen peroxide

Five drops tea tree oil

Instructions:

    1. Mix ingredients into a paste.

    2. Apply to surfaces and scrub with a sponge.

    3. Rinse clean.

Wood Furniture Polish

Ingredients:

1/4 cup olive oil

1/4 cup white vinegar

Ten drops lemon essential oil

Instructions:

    1. Combine ingredients in a spray bottle.

2. Shake well.

3. Apply to wooden furniture with a soft cloth and buff to shine.

Carpet Deodorizer

Ingredients:

One cup baking soda

Ten drops essential oil (lavender or citrus)

Instructions:

1. Mix baking soda and essential oil in a jar.

2. Sprinkle over carpets.

3. Let sit for 20 minutes, then vacuum.

Toilet Bowl Cleaner

Ingredients:

1/2 cup baking soda

1/4 cup white vinegar

Five drops tea tree oil

Instructions:

    1. Sprinkle baking soda in the toilet bowl.

    2. Add vinegar and essential oil.

    3. Scrub with a toilet brush and flush.

Dish Soap

Ingredients:

1/2 cup liquid castile soap

1/4 cup distilled water

One teaspoon olive oil

Ten drops lemon essential oil

Instructions:

    1. Combine all ingredients in a squeeze bottle.

    2. Shake well before each use.

3. Use like regular dish soap.

Laundry Detergent

Ingredients:

One bar unscented castile soap (grated)

One cup washing soda

One cup borax or baking soda

Instructions:

1. Mix grated soap, washing soda, and borax or baking soda in a container.

2. Store in an airtight container.

3. Use 1-2 tablespoons per load of laundry.

Oven Cleaner

Ingredients:

1/2 cup baking soda

Three tablespoons water

1/4 cup white vinegar (optional, for tough stains)

Instructions:

1. Mix baking soda and water into a paste.

2. Spread over oven surfaces and let sit overnight.

3. Wipe clean with a damp cloth. Spray vinegar and scrub for tough spots.

Non-Toxic Brass Cleaner

Ingredients:

1/2 lemon

One tablespoon baking soda

Instructions:

1. Sprinkle baking soda on the cut lemon.

2. Rub on brass and let sit for 5 minutes.

3. Rinse with water and buff with a soft cloth.

Cleaning Chopping Boards

Ingredients:

1/2 lemon

One tablespoon coarse salt

Instructions:

1. Sprinkle salt over the chopping board.

2. Scrub with the lemon.

3. Rinse clean and let air dry.

Disinfecting Wipes

Ingredients:

One cup distilled water

1/4 cup rubbing alcohol

Ten drops tea tree essential oil

Cloth squares or paper towels

Instructions:

    1. Mix water, alcohol, and essential oil in a bowl.

    2. Soak cloth squares or paper towels in the mixture.

    3. Store in an airtight container. Use as needed.

Clean Drains

Ingredients:

1/2 cup baking soda

1/2 cup white vinegar

Boiling water

Instructions:

    1. Pour baking soda into the drain, followed by vinegar.

    2. Let sit for 10 minutes.

3. Flush with boiling water.

Mattress Cleaner

Ingredients:

One cup baking soda

Ten drops lavender essential oil

Instructions:

1. Mix baking soda and lavender essential oil.

2. Sprinkle over the mattress.

3. Let sit for 30 minutes, then vacuum.

Non-Toxic Heavy-Duty Scrub

Ingredients:

1/2 cup baking soda

Two tablespoons coarse salt

One tablespoon liquid castile soap

Instructions:

    1. Mix ingredients into a paste.

    2. Use to scrub tough stains on pots, pans, or sinks.

    3. Rinse clean.

Chapter 26

Personal Care and Skincare Recipes

Magnesium Spray (Relaxation and Muscle Relief)

Ingredients:

1/2 cup magnesium chloride flakes

1/2 cup distilled water

Optional: 5-10 drops lavender or chamomile essential oil

Instructions:

1. Boil the distilled water and pour it into a glass bowl.

2. Add magnesium chloride flakes and stir until dissolved.

3. Let it cool and pour into a spray bottle.

4. Add essential oils if desired.

5. Spray on your skin (legs, arms, or feet) as needed for relaxation or muscle relief. A slight tingling sensation is normal.

DIY Lip Balm

Ingredients:

Two tablespoons beeswax pellets

Two tablespoons coconut oil

One tablespoon shea butter or cocoa butter

Five drops peppermint or vanilla essential oil (optional)

Instructions:

Melt beeswax, coconut oil, and shea butter in a double boiler.

Remove from heat and stir in essential oil.

Pour into small containers or tubes.

Let cool before use.

Natural Body Butter

Ingredients:

1/2 cup shea butter

1/4 cup coconut oil

1/4 cup almond or jojoba oil

10-15 drops essential oil (optional)

Instructions:

Melt shea butter and coconut oil in a double boiler.

Remove from heat and mix in almond oil.

Add essential oil and whip with a hand mixer until fluffy.

Store in a glass jar.

Non-Toxic Room Spray

Ingredients:

One cup distilled water

Two tablespoons vodka or rubbing alcohol

Ten drops essential oil (e.g., lemon, lavender, or eucalyptus)

Instructions:

Combine all ingredients in a spray bottle.

Shake well before use.

Spray around the home.

DIY Deodorant

Ingredients:

Two tablespoons coconut oil

Two tablespoons shea butter

Two tablespoons baking soda

Two tablespoons arrowroot powder or cornstarch

5-10 drops tea tree or lavender essential oil

Instructions:

Melt coconut oil and shea butter in a double boiler.

Remove from heat, stir in baking soda and arrowroot powder.

Add essential oil and pour into a jar or deodorant container.

Let harden before use.

Non-Toxic Toothpaste

Ingredients:

Two tablespoons coconut oil

One tablespoon baking soda

One teaspoon xylitol (optional, for sweetness)

Five drops peppermint essential oil

Instructions:

Mix all ingredients into a smooth paste.

Store in a small jar.

Use as regular toothpaste.

Natural Hand Scrub

Ingredients:

1/2 cup sugar or fine salt

1/4 cup coconut oil

Five drops essential oil (orange or mint)

Instructions:

    1. Mix sugar and coconut oil into a paste.

    2. Add essential oil and store in a jar.

    3. Use to exfoliate hands, then rinse with warm water.

DIY Hair Conditioner

Ingredients:

One cup distilled water

Two tablespoons apple cider vinegar

One teaspoon argan or jojoba oil

Five drops lavender or rosemary essential oil

Instructions:

    1. Combine all ingredients in a spray bottle.

    2. Shake before use.

    3. Spray onto damp hair. No rinsing needed.

Non-Toxic Essential Oil Shaving Cream

Ingredients:

1/4 cup shea butter

1/4 cup coconut oil

1/4 cup olive oil

Ten drops peppermint or lavender essential oil

Instructions:

1. Melt shea butter and coconut oil in a double boiler.

2. Add olive oil and essential oils.

3. Whip the mixture with a hand mixer.

Store in a jar and use as a shaving cream

DIY Face Balm

Ingredients:

1/4 cup shea butter

Two tablespoons coconut oil

One tablespoon rosehip oil

Five drops geranium essential oil (optional)

Instructions:

    1. Melt shea butter and coconut oil in a double boiler.

    2. Stir in rosehip oil and essential oils.

    3. Store in a jar. Use as a night balm.

Natural Body Scrub

Ingredients:

One cup sugar or salt

1/4 cup olive oil or coconut oil

Ten drops essential oil (lavender or citrus)

Instructions:

    1. Mix all ingredients in a bowl.

    2. Store in a jar.

    3. Use to exfoliate skin, then rinse.

Herbal Hair Care Shampoo

Ingredients:

1/4 cup liquid castile soap

1/4 cup aloe vera gel

One teaspoon jojoba oil

Ten drops rosemary essential oil

Instructions:

1. Mix all ingredients in a bottle.

2. Shake before each use.

3. Apply to wet hair, lather, and rinse.

Natural Lip Scrub

Ingredients:

One tablespoon sugar

One teaspoon honey

One teaspoon coconut oil

Instructions:

    1. Mix ingredients into a paste.

    2. Gently scrub onto lips.

    3. Rinse with warm water.

Natural Deodorizer Spray

Ingredients:

One cup distilled water

Two tablespoons vodka or rubbing alcohol

Ten drops tea tree oil

Five drops eucalyptus essential oil

Instructions:

    1. Mix ingredients in a spray bottle.

    2. Shake well.

    3. Spray in areas with odors, such as shoes or trash cans.

Face Wash for Acne

Ingredients:

Two tablespoons liquid castile soap

One teaspoon raw honey

One teaspoon aloe vera gel

Three drops tea tree oil

Instructions:

1. Mix all ingredients in a small bottle.

2. Use a pea-sized amount to cleanse your face daily.

Herbal Salve

Ingredients:

One cup infused herbal oil (e.g., calendula or comfrey)

1/4 cup beeswax

Optional: 10 drops tea tree oil (antimicrobial)

Instructions:

    1. Melt oil and beeswax in a double boiler.

    2. Remove from heat and stir in essential oil.

    3. Pour into tins and let cool.

Non-Toxic Essential Oil Hair Conditioner

Ingredients:

One cup distilled water

Two tablespoons apple cider vinegar

One teaspoon argan or coconut oil

Five drops lavender or rosemary essential oil

Instructions:

    1. Combine in a spray bottle.

    2. Spray on damp hair; no rinsing needed.

Non-Toxic Essential Oil Lip Balm

Ingredients:

Two tablespoons beeswax

Two tablespoons coconut oil

One tablespoon shea butter

Optional: 5 drops peppermint or vanilla essential oil

Instructions:

1. Melt beeswax, coconut oil, and shea butter in a double boiler.

2. Add essential oil, pour into lip balm tubes, and let cool.

Non-Toxic Essential Oil Body Wash

Ingredients:

1/2 cup liquid castile soap

1/4 cup honey

Two tablespoons coconut oil

Ten drops lavender or citrus essential oil

Instructions:

1. Mix in a bottle and shake before use.

Non-Toxic Whipped Lip Cream

Ingredients:

One tablespoon shea butter

One tablespoon coconut oil

1/2 teaspoon beeswax

Optional: 3 drops vanilla or peppermint essential oil

Instructions:

1. Melt shea butter, coconut oil, and beeswax in a double boiler.

2. Whip with a hand mixer until creamy.

3. Store in a small jar.

Chapter 27

Advanced Cleaning and Household Recipes

Laundry Bar Soap

Ingredients:

One cup grated castile soap

1/2 cup washing soda

1/2 cup borax (optional, or use baking soda for a gentler option)

Two tablespoons water

Instructions:

Melt grated castile soap in a saucepan with water over low heat.

1. Remove from heat, stir in washing soda and borax (or baking soda).

2. Pour into molds and let set for 24 hours.

3. Use as a stain remover or grate into laundry detergent.

Window and Stainless-Steel Cleaner

Ingredients:

One cup distilled water

1/4 cup white vinegar

One teaspoon cornstarch (for streak-free shine)

Five drops of lemon essential oil

Instructions:

1. Mix ingredients in a spray bottle.

2. Shake well before use. Spray onto windows or stainless steel, then wipe with a microfiber cloth.

Sleepy Time Magnesium Butter

Ingredients:

1/4 cup magnesium chloride flakes

1/4 cup warm water

1/2 cup shea butter

Two tablespoons coconut oil

Ten drops lavender essential oil

Instructions:

1. Dissolve magnesium flakes in warm water; let cool.

2. Melt shea butter and coconut oil in a double boiler.

3. Whip cooled magnesium water into the oils and add lavender oil.

4. Store in a jar and apply to feet or body before bedtime.

Homemade Infused Lavender Oil

Ingredients:

One cup dried lavender flowers

One cup carrier oil (e.g., almond, olive, or jojoba)

Instructions:

1. Place lavender flowers in a jar and cover with oil.

2. Seal tightly and let sit in a sunny spot for 2 weeks.

3. Strain into a clean jar. Use for massages, skin care, or aromatherapy.

Odor Eliminator Spray

Ingredients:

One cup distilled water

Two tablespoons vodka or rubbing alcohol

Ten drops tea tree oil

Ten drops eucalyptus or lemon essential oil

Instructions:

1. Mix all ingredients in a spray bottle.

2. Shake well and spray in smelly areas (shoes, trash cans, etc.).

Herbal Linen Spray

Ingredients:

One cup distilled water

Two tablespoons vodka or rubbing alcohol

Ten drops lavender essential oil

Five drops chamomile or eucalyptus essential oil

Instructions:

1. Mix in a spray bottle.

2. Shake and lightly mist on linens for a calming scent.

Disinfecting Spray

Ingredients:

One cup distilled water

1/2 cup rubbing alcohol

Ten drops eucalyptus essential oil

Instructions:

1. Combine all ingredients in a spray bottle.

2. Shake well before use.

3. Spray on surfaces to disinfect.

Toilet Cleaning Tablets

Ingredients:

One cup baking soda

1/4 cup citric acid

Ten drops tea tree oil

Water (just enough to form a paste)

Instructions:

    1. Mix baking soda and citric acid in a bowl.

    2. Add water slowly until the mixture holds together.

    3. Press into molds and let dry overnight.

    4. Drop one tablet into the toilet as needed.

Non-Toxic Wall and Ceiling Cleaner

Ingredients:

One gallon warm water

1/4 cup white vinegar

Five drops lavender essential oil (optional)

Instructions:

    1. Mix all ingredients in a bucket.

    2. Use a microfiber cloth or mop to clean walls and ceilings.

Non-Toxic Heavy-Duty Scrub

Ingredients:

1/2 cup baking soda

Two tablespoons coarse salt

One tablespoon liquid castile soap

Instructions:

1. Mix ingredients into a paste.

2. Use to scrub tough stains on pots, pans, or sinks.

3. Rinse clean.

Rug and Carpet Cleaner

Ingredients:

One cup baking soda

1/4 cup cornstarch

Ten drops lemon essential oil

Instructions:

1. Mix ingredients in a container.

2. Sprinkle over rugs or carpets.

3. Let sit for 20 minutes, then vacuum.

Non-Toxic Kitchen Cleaner and Deodorizer

Ingredients:

1/4 cup baking soda

1/4 cup white vinegar

Ten drops tea tree or lemon essential oil

Instructions:

1. Apply baking soda to kitchen surfaces.

2. Spray with vinegar and essential oil solution.

3. Wipe clean with a cloth.

Magical Sink Scrub

Ingredients:

1/2 cup baking soda

1/4 cup fine salt

One tablespoon eco-friendly dish soap

Five drops lemon essential oil

Instructions:

1. Mix ingredients into a paste.

2. Apply to the sink and scrub with a sponge.

3. Rinse clean.

Homemade Laundry Detergent

Ingredients:

One cup washing soda

One cup borax (or baking soda)

One bar grated castile soap

Optional: 10 drops lavender or citrus essential oil

Instructions:

    1. Mix ingredients in a container.

    2. Use 1-2 tablespoons per load.

Dishwasher Detergent

Ingredients:

One cup washing soda

One cup baking soda

1/2 cup citric acid

1/2 cup coarse salt

Instructions:

    1. Mix ingredients and store in an airtight container.

    2. Use 1 tablespoon per dishwasher load.

Non-Toxic Rinse Aid for Dishwasher

Ingredients:

One cup white vinegar

Ten drops lemon essential oil

Instructions:

    1. Add to the rinse aid compartment of your dishwasher.

Non-Toxic Dishwasher Tablets

Ingredients:

One cup washing soda

One cup baking soda

1/2 cup citric acid

1/2 cup coarse salt

Water (just enough to form tablets)

Instructions:

    1. Mix ingredients and add water slowly until the mixture holds together.

    2. Press into molds and let dry for 24 hours.

Non-Toxic Essential Oil Herbal Laundry Wash

Ingredients:

One cup washing soda

One cup baking soda

One bar grated castile soap

Ten drops lavender or lemon essential oil

Instructions:

1. Mix and store in an airtight container.

2. Use 1-2 tablespoons per load.

Non-Toxic Essential Oil Herbal Laundry Softener

Ingredients:

One cup white vinegar

Ten drops lavender or eucalyptus essential oil

Instructions:

1. Add to the fabric softener compartment of your washing machine.

Non-Toxic Laundry Wash for Sensitive Skin

Ingredients:

One cup washing soda

One cup baking soda

One bar grated unscented castile soap

Instructions:

1. Mix and store in an airtight container.

2. Use 1 tablespoon per load.

Non-Toxic Herbal Stain Remover

Ingredients:

1/4 cup baking soda

1/4 cup white vinegar

Five drops lemon essential oil

Instructions:

1. Mix into a paste and apply to stains.

2. Let sit for 30 minutes, then wash.

Non-Toxic Hand Wash

Ingredients:

1/2 cup liquid castile soap

1/2 cup distilled water

Five drops lavender essential oil

Instructions:

    1. Combine in a soap dispenser.

    2. Shake before use.

Non-Toxic Dish Wash

Ingredients:

1/2 cup liquid castile soap

1/4 cup distilled water

One teaspoon olive oil

Ten drops lemon essential oil

Instructions:

    1. Mix in a bottle.

    2. Shake before use.

Non-Toxic Weed Killer

Ingredients:

One gallon white vinegar

1/2 cup salt

One tablespoon dish soap

Instructions:

1. Mix ingredients in a spray bottle.

2. Spray directly onto weeds.

Non-Toxic Oven and Stove Solutions

Ingredients:

1/2 cup baking soda

Two tablespoons water

Optional: 1 tablespoon white vinegar for tough stains

Instructions:

    1. Mix baking soda and water into a paste.

    2. Spread on oven surfaces and let sit overnight.

    3. Wipe clean with a damp cloth.

Non-Toxic Home Appliance Cleaner

Ingredients:

1/4 cup baking soda

1/4 cup white vinegar

Instructions:

    1. Apply baking soda to appliance surfaces.

    2. Spray with vinegar and wipe clean.

Non-Toxic Floor Cleaning

Ingredients:

One gallon warm water

1/2 cup white vinegar

Five drops eucalyptus essential oil

Instructions:

1. Mix in a mop bucket.

2. Mop floors as usual.

Keeping Your Home Smelling Clean and Fresh

Ingredients:

One cup distilled water

Two tablespoons vodka

Ten drops lavender or citrus essential oil

Instructions:

1. Combine in a spray bottle.

2. Mist in rooms as needed.

Gentle Marble Cleaning

Ingredients:

1/4 cup mild dish soap

One gallon warm water

Instructions:

1. Mix and use a soft sponge to clean marble surfaces.

2. Rinse with clean water and dry with a soft cloth.

3. Avoid vinegar, lemon, or abrasive cleaners to prevent etching.

Chapter 28

Lifestyle and General Wellness

Keeping Laundry Whites Bright

Ingredients:

1/2 cup baking soda

1/2 cup hydrogen peroxide

One gallon warm water

Instructions:

Soak white clothes in the solution for 30 minutes.

Wash as usual. Add 1/4 cup white vinegar to the rinse cycle for brightness.

Cleaning Armpit Stains

Ingredients:

1/4 cup baking soda

One tablespoon hydrogen peroxide

One tablespoon dish soap

Instructions:

> 1. Mix into a paste and apply to stains.

> 2. Let sit for 30 minutes, then wash as usual.

Cleaning Grout and Shower Screens

Ingredients:

1/2 cup baking soda

1/4 cup white vinegar

Optional: 5 drops tea tree oil (antifungal)

Instructions:

1. Sprinkle baking soda on grout or screens.

2. Spray with vinegar and scrub with a brush or sponge.

3. Rinse with water.

Steam Cleaner and Squeegee for Cleaner Windows

Instructions:

Use distilled water in the steam cleaner to avoid streaks.

1. Steam the windows and use a squeegee to wipe clean immediately.

2. Finish with a microfiber cloth for a polished shine

Tincture Recipes

Ingredients:

One part dried herbs (e.g., echinacea, chamomile, or valerian)

Three parts high-proof alcohol (e.g., vodka)

Instructions:

Combine herbs and alcohol in a jar.

Seal and store in a cool, dark place for 4-6 weeks, shaking occasionally.

Strain and store in a dark glass bottle.

Non-Toxic Vapour Rub

Ingredients:

1/4 cup coconut oil

One tablespoon beeswax

Ten drops eucalyptus oil

Five drops peppermint oil

Instructions:

1. Melt coconut oil and beeswax in a double boiler.//
2. Remove from heat, add essential oils, and store in a jar.

Whipped Tallow Balm

Ingredients:

1/2 cup grass-fed tallow

Two tablespoons olive oil or jojoba oil

Ten drops lavender or chamomile essential oil (optional)

Instructions:

1. Melt tallow in a double boiler.

2. Let cool until semi-solid.

3. Whip with a hand mixer while adding olive oil and essential oils.

4. Store in a jar and use as a moisturizer.

Conquer Bug Season: Bug Spray

Ingredients:

1/2 cup witch hazel

1/2 cup distilled water

Ten drops citronella oil

Ten drops eucalyptus oil

Five drops lavender or peppermint oil

Instructions:

    1. Combine all ingredients in a spray bottle.

    2. Shake well before use.

    3. Spray on exposed skin.

Herbal Sleepy-Time Magnesium Butter

Ingredients:

1/4 cup magnesium chloride flakes

1/4 cup warm water

1/2 cup shea butter

Two tablespoons coconut oil

Ten drops lavender essential oil

Instructions:

    1. Dissolve magnesium flakes in warm water and let cool.

    2. Melt shea butter and coconut oil in a double boiler.

    3. Mix magnesium water into the oils.

4. Add lavender oil and whip until fluffy.

5. Store in a jar. Apply to feet or body before bed.

Immune-Boosting Tincture

Ingredients:

One part echinacea and elderberry

Three parts high-proof alcohol (vodka)

Instructions:

1. Combine herbs and alcohol in a jar.

2. Seal and store for 4-6 weeks, shaking occasionally.

3. Strain and store in a dark glass bottle. Use 1-2 drops as needed.

Natural Energy Boost Tea

Ingredients:

One teaspoon green tea leaves

One teaspoon dried ginger

One cup hot water

Honey to taste

Instructions:

1. Combine green tea and ginger in a teapot.

2. Add hot water and let steep for 5 minutes.

3. Strain and add honey if desired.

Chapter 29

Conclusion

In this book, we explored different elements of establishing a healthy, non-toxic home. Let's summarize the essential insights and motivate you to embark on the journey of incorporating these practices into your living space.

Key Takeaways:

Understanding Toxins in the Home: We uncovered the sources of common indoor pollutants, their health impacts, and strategies to minimize exposure. Recognizing and addressing these toxins is crucial for fostering a healthier indoor environment.

Building a Non-Toxic Home Environment: We've highlighted ways to create a safe and sustainable home, from selecting eco-friendly building materials to enhancing indoor air quality, reducing electromagnetic field exposure, and preventing mold growth.

Natural Cleaning and Maintenance: We explored the benefits of using natural cleaning agents like vinegar, baking soda, and essential oils. You can maintain a clean, chemical-free home by incorporating these into regular cleaning routines.

Adopting Sustainable Living Practices: Implementing energy-efficient habits, reducing waste, conserving water, and embracing eco-friendly choices are foundational to sustainable living. These practices benefit the planet and support healthier lifestyles.

Encouragement to Act:

Now that you understand these principles comprehensively, it's time to bring them to life. Transforming your home into a non-toxic, healthy space is a rewarding journey that starts with small, intentional changes. Gradually adopt sustainable habits and make informed choices that align with your goals. No matter how small, every effort contributes to a safer, healthier, and more sustainable environment for you, your family, and the planet.

References

Books and Publications

Berry, Wendell. The Unsettling of America: Culture and Agriculture. San Francisco: Sierra Club Books, 1977.

Johnson, Bea. *Zero Waste Home: The Ultimate Guide to Simplifying Your Life by Reducing Your Waste.* New York: Scribner, 2013.

Siegel-Maier, Karyn. *The Naturally Clean Home: 150 Super-Easy Herbal Formulas for Green Cleaning.* North Adams: Storey Publishing, 2008.

Swift, Katja, and Ryn Midura. *Herbal Medicine for Beginners: Your Guide to Healing Common Ailments with 35 Medicinal Herbs.* Emeryville: Callisto Media, 2018.

Howard, Brian. *The Green Home: Creating a Healthy, Environmentally Friendly, and Sustainable Living Space.* Chicago: Agate Publishing, 2011.

Crinnion, Walter J. *Clean, Green, and Lean: Get Rid of the Toxins That Make You Fat.* Hoboken: Wiley, 2010.

Weinstein, Annie Berthold-Bond. *Better Basics for the Home: Simple Solutions for Less Toxic Living.* New York: Three Rivers Press, 1999.

Websites and Online Resources

Environmental Working Group. "EWG's Guide to Healthy Cleaning." https://www.ewg.org.

ENERGY STAR. "Energy Efficiency at Home." U.S. Environmental Protection Agency. https://www.energystar.gov.

Green Seal. "Standards and Certification." https://www.greenseal.org

Wellness Mama. "DIY Cleaning and Personal Care Recipes." https://wellnessmama.com

Mountain Rose Herbs Blog. "Herbal Recipes and Remedies." https://blog.mountainroseherbs.com

U.S. Environmental Protection Agency. "Indoor Air Quality." https://www.epa.gov/indoor-air-quality-iaq

Forest Stewardship Council. "Certification and Standards." https://www.fsc.org

Scientific and Research-Based Articles

National Institute of Environmental Health Sciences. "Indoor Air Quality: Understanding Common Pollutants."

U.S. Environmental Protection Agency (EPA). "Volatile Organic Compounds' Impact on Indoor Air Quality."

American Lung Association. "The Impact of Poor Indoor Air Quality on Health."

National Resources Defense Council (NRDC). "How to Reduce Exposure to Household Chemicals."

Certifications and Guidelines

ENERGY STAR. "Certified Products for Energy Efficiency."

USDA. "Organic Certification Standards."

Green Seal. "The Environmental Standard for Cleaning Products."

Cradle to Cradle Products Innovation Institute. "Cradle to Cradle Certification Program." https://www.c2ccertified.org

WaterSense. "Water Efficiency Certification." https://www.epa.gov/watersense

Tools and Products Mentioned

HEPA Air Purifiers. "Recommended Brands for Improved Indoor Air Quality."

Castile Soap. "Eco-Friendly Cleaning Ingredients for Home and Personal Care."

Bamboo Flooring. "Durable and Renewable Building Materials."

Compost Bins. "Efficient Systems for Organic Waste Recycling."

Reusable Household Items. "Alternatives to Single-Use Plastics."

Online Courses and Learning Resources

Herbal Academy. "Foundations of Herbalism." https://theherbalacademy.com

Coursera. "Sustainable Living Practices." https://www.coursera.org

Skillshare. "DIY Natural Cleaning Products." https://www.skillshare.com

Acknowledgments

Special thanks to the Environmental Working Group, Green Seal, and the U.S. Environmental Protection Agency for their dedication to promoting non-toxic and sustainable living practices. Additional gratitude to herbalists and sustainable living advocates worldwide for their continued efforts to inspire healthier, greener lifestyles.

www.ingramcontent.com/pod-product-compliance
Lightning Source LLC
Chambersburg PA
CBHW060604080526
44585CB00013B/678